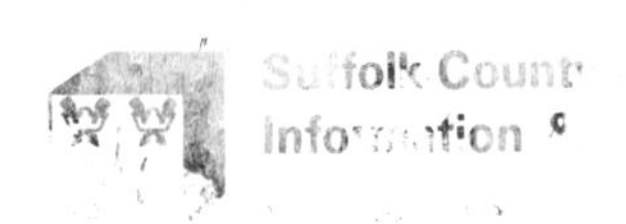

Adrian Mindel was born in South
University of the Witwatersrand fr
1973. He has been a Senior Lecture
in Genito-Urinary Medicine at the University College and Middlesex School of Medicine since 1983. He has been involved in research in genital herpes since 1980 and has a particular interest in the treatment of the condition, running a special weekly 'herpes clinic' at the Middlesex Hospital. He has also written numerous articles and medical text books.

Orla Carney graduated in English Literature from Newcastle University and then joined the nursing profession, qualifying in 1985. She concentrated on well women and family planning work, which she still practises. Since 1987 she has worked as research nurse specialising in genital herpes, in the Genito-Urinary clinic of the Middlesex Hospital. Her main interests at work are psychological aspects of the infection, and counselling.

OPTIMA

HERPES

What it is and how to cope

Adrian Mindel MRCP
and Orla Carney RGN

Illustrated by
Maggie Raynor

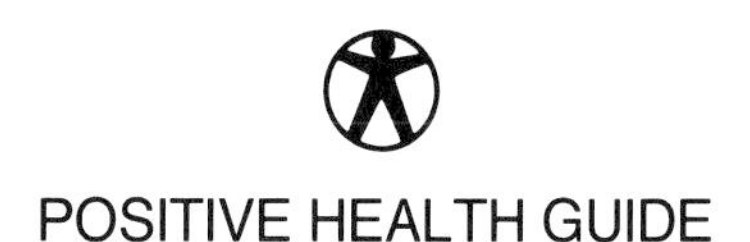

POSITIVE HEALTH GUIDE

First published in 1991 by
Macdonald Optima, a division of
Macdonald & Co. (Publishers) Ltd

A member of Maxwell Macmillan Pergamon Publishing Corporation plc

British Library Cataloguing in Publication Data
Mindel, Adrian, 1949-
1. Man. Herpes simplex
I. Title II. Carney, Orla III. Series

ISBN 0-356-18687-3

Macdonald & Co. (Publishers) Ltd
Orbit House
1 New Fetter Lane
London EC4A 1AR

Typeset in Times by Leaper & Gard Ltd, Bristol

Printed and bound in Great Britain by
BPCC Hazell Books
Aylesbury, Bucks, England
Member of BPCC Ltd.

CONTENTS

PREFACE

Genital herpes is an extremely common infection, and whilst for most individuals it is an occasional nuisance, for a few it is a chronic and psychologically disabling condition. In the late 1970s and early 1980s herpes was a popular 'media' disease, many of the newspaper and magazine reports appearing at that time were inaccurate and sensational and caused distress to many people; and many of the myths and misconceptions concerning the illness are still common.

The object of this book is to give people with herpes the facts in an up-to-date, accurate and non-sensational way. Areas covered include what causes herpes, its transmission, the clinical features, diagnosis and treatment, associated problems, psychological response to the infection, self help and where to go if you need advice on treatment.

The book is aimed primarily at people who have genital herpes but we hope it will also be of interest to partners, friends and family as well as to doctors, nurses, health advisors and counsellors who may see people with the infection.

ACKNOWLEDGEMENTS

We would like to thank the following for their help, Katerina Ayres, Claire Wilson, Paula Williams, our editor Harriet Griffey and all the patients with genital herpes who have participated in clinical trials and studies at The Middlesex Hospital over the past ten years.

1

THE VIRUS AND ITS TRANSMISSION

Genital herpes is caused by a virus called the *Herpes simplex* virus (HSV). There are two *Herpes simplex* viruses, designated HSV type 1 and HSV type 2, and both can cause genital herpes.

Herpes Simplex viruses belong to a group of viruses called the human herpes viruses. Other members of the group include:

- *Varicella zoster*, the cause of chickenpox and shingles.
- The Epstein-Barr virus, the cause of glandular fever.
- Cytomegalovirus (CMV), another virus occasionally causing a glandular-fever-like illness.
- And a recently described virus called the human herpes virus 6 (HHV6) whose role in disease production (if any) remains unknown.

THE VIRUS

A virus is a minute microorganism, so small that it cannot be seen with an ordinary microscope, although it can be seen with an electron microscope. Viruses contain RNA (ribonucleic acid) or DNA (deoxyribonucleic acid); these are complex chemicals containing the genetic (inheritable) material. *Herpes simplex* virus contains DNA, enclosed within a rigid structure or box, called the capsid, which is then surrounded by a membrane or envelope. On the surface of the envelope are a number of complex structures called glycoproteins (a glycoprotein is a mixture of sugars and proteins) which are important in allowing the virus to attach to human cells. These glycoproteins are also important in stimulating the body's immune responses (discussed below).

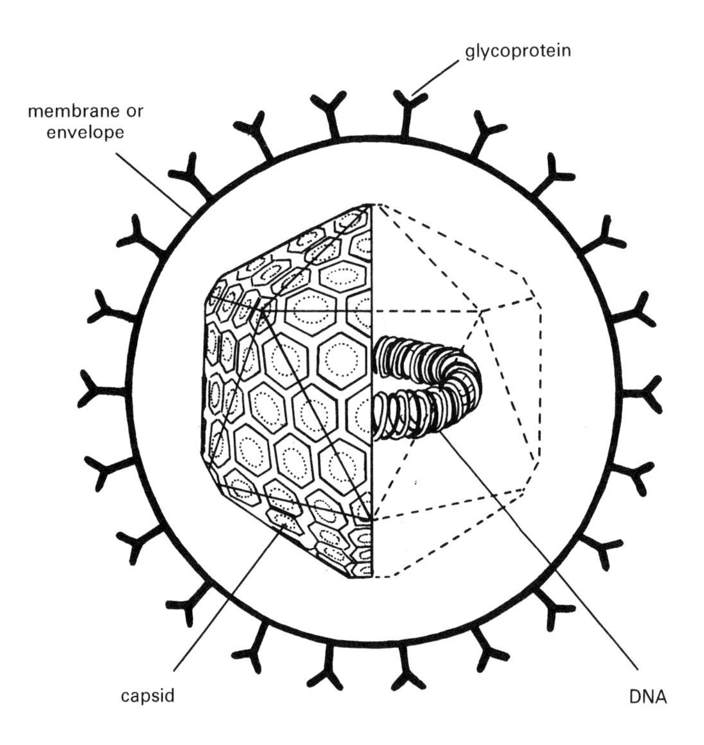

Structure of *Herpes simplex* virus.

HSV enters the body via the cells of the skin or the mucous membranes (the lining of the inside of the mouth or genitals); these cells are called epithelial cells. First the virus attaches to the surface of the cells, the envelope is detached and the capsid containing the DNA enters the cells. The capsid is then removed and the viral DNA takes over the control of the epithelial cell, reorganising the functions of the cell so that they produce a new batch of viruses; in this way the virus reproduces itself. The new viral particles then leave the epithelial cell and move on to infect adjoining cells, the infected epithelial cell ultimately dying. It is the death of these epithelial cells that causes the blisters and sores typical of herpes (see Chapter 2).

HSV types 1 and 2

The two *Herpes simplex* viruses, HSV 1 and HSV 2, are very similar. The genetic composition of the two viruses, i.e. the DNA, shows some differences, and some of the glycoproteins on the outer surface of the envelope are also unique to each virus; otherwise the two viruses are identical.

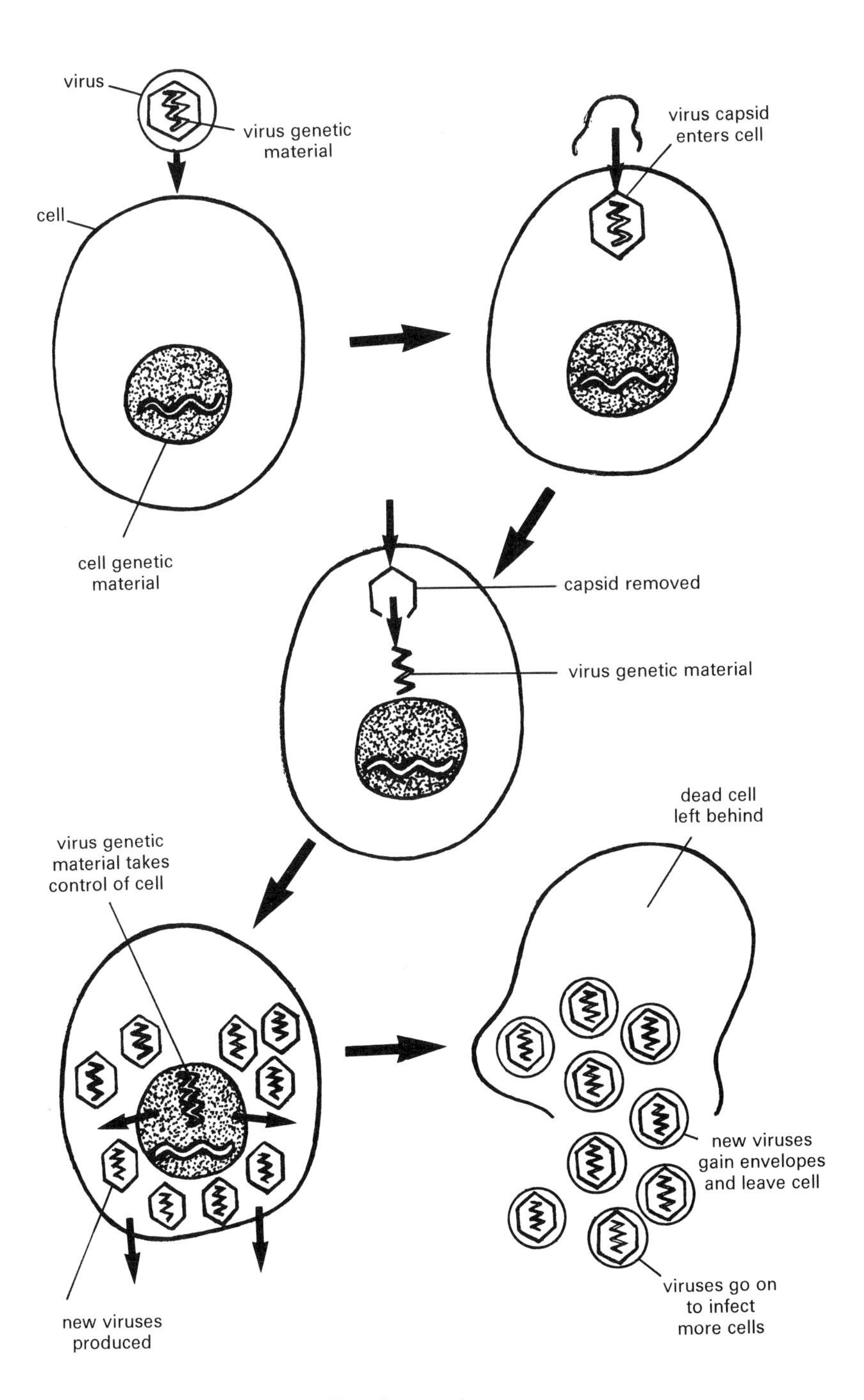

How herpes infects a cell and reproduces.

Both HSV type 1 and type 2 can cause genital herpes. Type 1 infection is usually transmitted via orogenital sex and type 2 by vaginal or anal sex. The percentage of genital infections caused by HSV 1 is extremely variable, ranging from 0–60 per cent, these differences probably reflecting the variable popularity of orogenital sex in different communities.

The infection caused by the two viruses is indistinguishable. However, studies have shown that patients with HSV 2 infections are more likely to have frequent recurrences than those with HSV 1.

LATENCY AND REACTIVATION

Most human viruses are eliminated from the body by the immune system (discussed below). However, in the case of herpes this does not occur; instead the virus escapes the body's defences by migrating up the nerves to eventually live in nerve cells. In the case of genital herpes these nerve cells are at the base of the spine and are called the sacral ganglia; with oral herpes or cold sores these are near the ear and are called the trigeminal ganglia.

Herpes viruses in the nerves are inactive (latent) and do not cause any damage to the nerves. However, from time to time the virus may become active again, move back down the nerves and cause the recurrence of herpes where the nerve endings reach the skin and mucous membranes. The precise mechanisms involved in the establishment of latency and subsequent reactivation are not fully understood, although it is now known that a complex interrelationship exists between the virus, the infected nerve cells and the immune system of the infected individual.

Some factors that may lead to reactivation of the virus include the following:

- Local trauma to the skin or mucous membranes, associated with sexual intercourse or masturbation. The reason for this is thought to be due to minor damage caused to the nerve endings in the skin leading to stimulation of the nerves and reactivation of the virus within the nerve cells. As mentioned above, the virus then moves down the nerves to cause a recurrence.
- Menstruation, probably due to hormonal changes and local trauma.
- Type of virus. As mentioned above there are two HSV

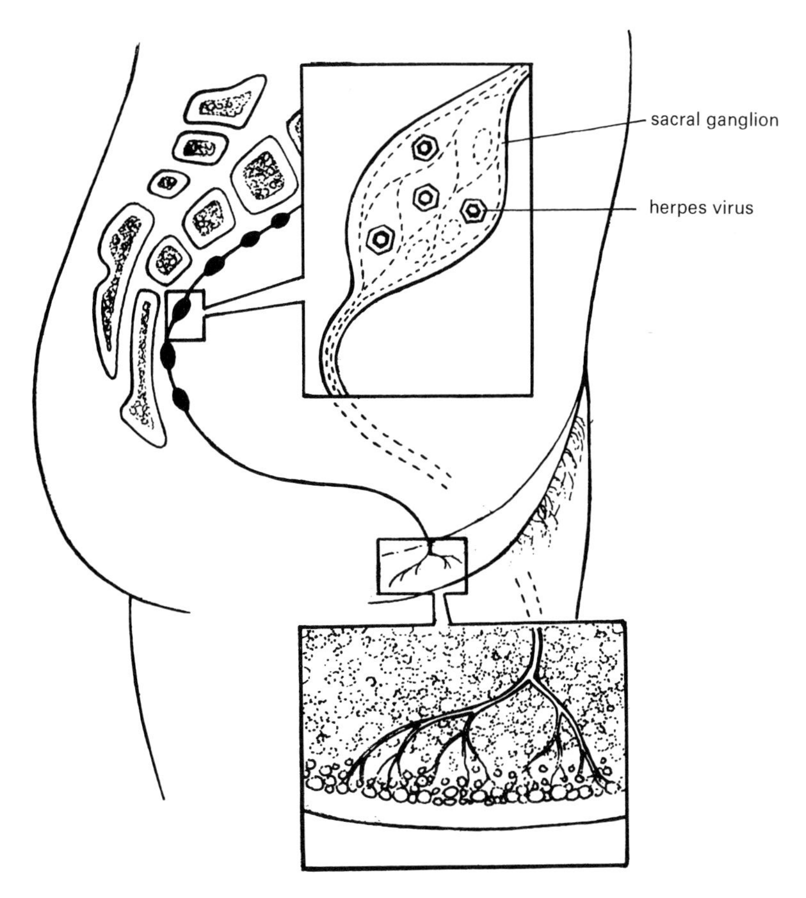

Latent herpes infection in sacral ganglion of nerves that supply sensation to the originally infected areas of skin.

viruses, designated HSV 1 and HSV 2. Both can cause genital herpes. HSV 2 infection of the genitals recurs more often than HSV 1 infection, although again the reasons for this are unclear.

- Other infections or general ill health and stress. Many people who have recurrent genital herpes find the outbreaks are more likely to occur during periods of ill health or at times of stress. Again, the reasons for this are unclear, but may be due to a minor temporary lowering of the body's immune defences. It is of some interest that recent research has suggested that stress may directly decrease the body's immune defences, possibly allowing recurrences to occur.

How often do recurrences occur?

When a person contracts genital herpes one of the questions that is usually asked is 'how often will the infection recur?' Unfortunately, there is no way of predicting this at the outset. Some people will never have a recurrence, whilst others will have very frequent outbreaks. In some the attacks become less frequent over a period of years, in others they remain the same. Many find that the frequency is variable – at some times the recurrences occur frequently, followed by prolonged periods when there are none or very few.

THE BODY'S DEFENCES

The body has a considerable array of defence mechanisms it can bring into play against the infective agents – bacteria, viruses, fungi and protozoa – that it comes up against.

Non-specific defences

The first line of defence is the skin. Intact skin is probably impermeable to most infective agents, including herpes, but damaged or abraded skin or mucosal surfaces do allow viral entry.

The second line of defence involves cells of the immune system. Three types of cells are involved, called neutrophils, macrophages and natural killer cells.

- The macrophages ingest (gobble up) infective agents, including herpes, and release a chemical called interferon which slows or stops the spread of the virus from one cell to another. Macrophages are also essential for the subsequent activation of other parts of immune response (discussed in detail below).
- Neutrophils ingest and then digest viruses.
- Natural killer cells, as their name implies, control the infection by destroying the body's cells that are infected.

Specific defences

The mechanisms mentioned above are all non-specific, i.e. they are involved in the control of many infections, not just herpes. In addition to these non-specific mechanisms, the body also produces specific responses to specific infecting agents such as herpes. There are two types of specific response:

- Cellular immunity, involving immune cells called lymphocytes.
- And humoral immunity, involving the production of complex proteins called antibodies.

The cellular immune response is activated following exposure to the virus. As its name implies, this aspect of the immune system involves the activation of various immune cells. The first step occurs when the virus is ingested by macrophages (see above). This results in release of chemicals called cytokines, which in turn activate cells called T lymphocytes. The T lymphocytes then attack and destroy other cells infected with the virus (see diagram on next page). Subsequently, when people have recurrences of herpes it is these same T lymphocytes that control the severity of the attack, again by destroying infected cells in the body. However, if the body's immune system is under severe pressure, e.g. during serious infection such as pneumonia, or is damaged, e.g. due to cancer or infection with the human immunodeficiency virus (HIV), the T lymphocytes do not operate efficiently and recurrences of herpes may become more prolonged, severe and frequent.

The humoral aspect of the immune system involves the production of chemicals called antibodies. Antibodies are complex proteins produced by cells called B lymphocytes. Antibodies are produced in response to all infections, and each antibody is specific for each infection. Antibodies coat infected cells allowing them to be destroyed by T lymphocytes and macrophages (see above). Antibodies are also important in preventing people becoming reinfected with certain viruses; for example, once an individual has had an infection such as chickenpox or mumps, antibodies prevent them getting the infection again. Unfortunately, herpes antibodies are an exception, in that they do not prevent reinfection; they just make it less likely to occur, and if it does occur the new infection is usually less severe. Herpes antibodies are also important in terminating each recurrence of the disease; without these antibodies recurrences would probably take a considerable time to heal.

The two *Herpes simplex* viruses, types 1 and 2, each produce different antibodies. However, because the viruses are so similar the antibodies produced are also similar. In practical terms this means that if people who have previously had cold sores, e.g. due to HSV 1, subsequently come into genital contact with HSV 2 they are less likely to develop genital herpes, and if they do the infection is usually less severe. And

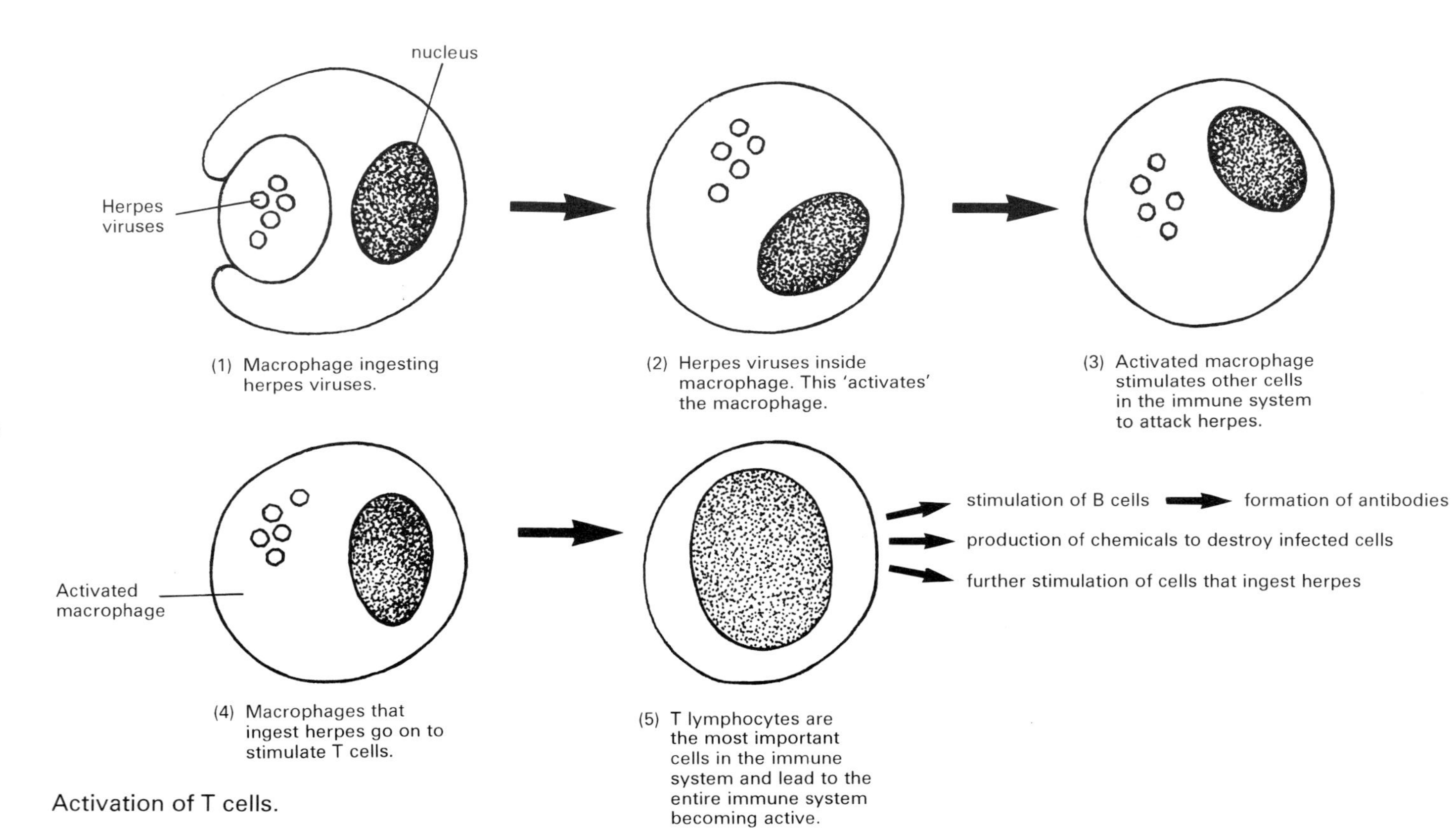

Activation of T cells.

the opposite is also true – people with previous genital herpes who come into contact with oral herpes are less likely to develop cold sores, and if they do the infection is less severe.

TRANSMISSION

Genital herpes is contracted following close personal contact with somebody who has the infection. Such contact may occur during vaginal intercourse (genital to genital contact), anal intercourse (genital to anal contact), orogenital sex (mouth to genital contact) or oroanal sex (mouth to anal contact). It is not contracted from towels, facecloths or toilets, nor is there any evidence that people with cold sores can infect their own genitals with herpes (or vice versa).

Transmission occurring from individuals with obvious clinical herpes, i.e. cold sores or genital herpes, is well documented, although most patients with active cold sores or genital herpes are usually aware of the infectious nature of their complaint and the majority probably avoid contact at that time. But many people who transmit herpes do not know that they themselves are infected with the virus; some people with the infection have no symptoms whatsoever, while others have minor problems, e.g. transient patches of redness, or small ulcers, which they do not recognise as being genital herpes. It is also not widely appreciated that people with active cold sores can transmit the infection during orogenital sex; as a consequence it is not at all unusual for someone within a monogamous relationship to develop genital herpes, even when the relationship has lasted many years. Sometimes the infection occurs because the couple have recently changed their sexual behaviour, e.g. started having orogenital sex for the first time.

If you have recently contracted herpes, it does not necessarily mean that your partner has been unfaithful, nor that he or she was aware that they themselves had the infection. So how is the virus transmitted from such people who have no signs or symptoms of the infection? The answer is that infectious viruses may be shed from the skin or mucous membranes, even if no obvious sores are present. Studies have shown that some of these people only have sores visible with a powerful magnifying glass, whilst in others the skin and mucous membranes are entirely normal.

The incubation period, i.e. the time from exposure until the first signs of the infection occur, is anything from two days to two weeks. It is not known how many people exposed to the virus actually develop the infection.

HOW COMMON IS GENITAL HERPES?

Genital herpes is a very common infection. In the developed world it is said to be the commonest cause of ulcers or sores of the genitals. However, in the developing world tropical sexually transmitted infections are more common.

In 1972 almost 5,000 cases of genital herpes were diagnosed from sexually transmitted disease (STD) clinics in the UK. Then, during the 1970s and early 1980s there was a dramatic increase in the number of cases seen, reaching a peak in 1985 with over 20,000 cases. Since then the number of people with herpes seen in clinics has decreased, perhaps reflecting increased condom usage as a consequence of the AIDS epidemic.

However, many patients with genital herpes do not attend STD clinics; some will go to their general practitioners, some to gynaecologists or to dermatologists. And many will not attend a doctor at all. As a consequence of this the total number of

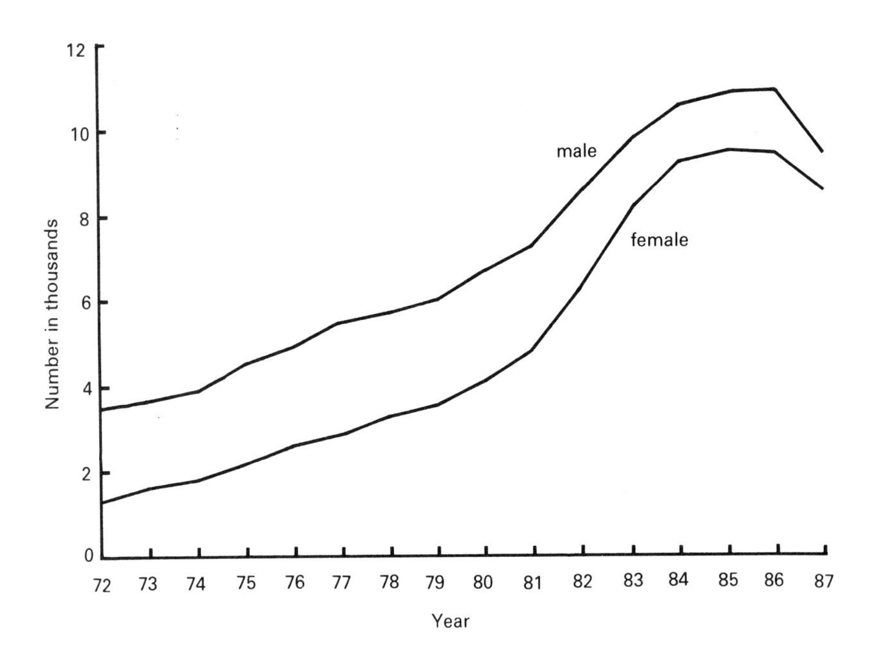

Incidence of herpes in the UK, 1972–87.

people with genital herpes in the UK is unknown, but at the very least it is likely to be many tens of thousands.

In the United States no accurate national data are available. However, herpes is said to be one of the most common sexually transmitted diseases. Estimates in the popular press have put the number of people infected with genital herpes at between 2 and 20 million. The Centers for Disease Control (CDC), a government-based agency in Atlanta, have estimated that there are between 300,000 and 500,000 new cases of herpes each year in the USA, and a recent survey suggested that as many as 25 million Americans may have been exposed to HSV type 2. Information from other Western countries is scarce, although herpes does seem to be a common infection.

The reasons for the dramatic increase in the number of people worldwide with genital herpes from the late 1960s to the early 1980s reflects greater sexual freedom and experimentation, decreased use of the condom (with increased use of the pill) and a greater mobility in society, particularly amongst young people. Over recent years there has been a slight decrease in the number of new patients with genital herpes, perhaps reflecting an increased awareness about safer sex and, as mentioned above, increased use of condoms following widespread publicity about the danger of infection with the human immunodeficiency virus (HIV) and AIDS.

The numbers of people with herpes mentioned above all represent clinical herpes, i.e. herpes which is apparent to both the patient and the doctor. But, as we saw above, if you are exposed to an infectious agent such as the herpes virus, your immune system produces antibodies specific to that infectious agent; so if antibodies to that infectious agent can be detected in your body, it means that you must have been infected with it at some time, even if you were not aware of it at the time. Studies looking at antibodies to herpes suggest that a large number of people have been exposed to the infection at some time in their lives, even though they did not have the classical clinical features of herpes (discussed in Chapter 2). These studies suggest that the true number of people with herpes, i.e. both clinical and inapparent, is substantially larger than we originally believed. Individuals with inapparent herpes are probably the source of new infection in many patients (see section on transmission above).

2

CLINICAL FEATURES

In most people the first episode of genital herpes is a severe illness lasting several weeks. However, the severity is extremely variable and in some it may be a very minor illness, often dismissed by the patient as an insignificant scratch, cut or abrasion. The most severe and prolonged infections occur in those who have never been exposed to the *Herpes simplex* virus before, whereas those who have, e.g. people with cold sores, tend to have a milder and shorter illness. Following healing of the first attack, many people have recurrences. In some they are frequent, in most they are occasional and in a fortunate few there are no further outbreaks.

The clinical features of primary and recurrent genital herpes and the characteristics of primary herpes in men and women are all a little different and each will be considered separately.

WOMEN

The first attack of genital herpes occurs two to fourteen days after exposure to an infected partner. Pain in the genital area, pain on urination and feeling as if one has flu (fevers, aches in the joints and muscles, and general feeling of ill health) are usually the first symptoms.

Over the next two to seven days the symptoms often get progressively worse. Painful swellings in the groin may be noticed, due to inflammation of the lymph glands. The lymph glands are found throughout the body and are part of the body's immune system (see Chapter 1), and they are often swollen and tender in response to infection, e.g. swollen glands in the neck when one has a sore throat. This is because the lymph nodes are packed with immunologically active cells; if there is an infection nearby, these cells have to work hard

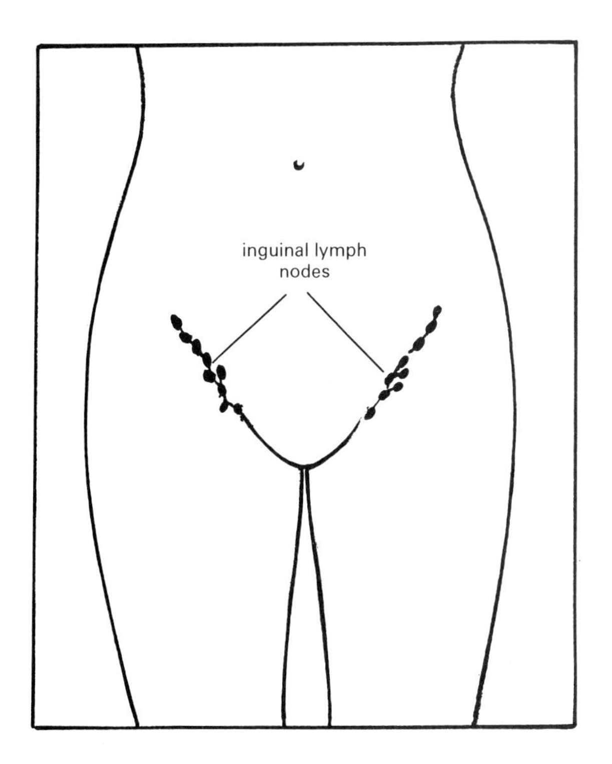

Location of the inguinal lymph nodes in the groin.

combating the infection and dealing with infected cells. This is why they swell and become tender.

A vaginal discharge may also occur. This is due to inflammation of the cervix (the neck of the womb) because of infection of the cervix with herpes. Herpes infection of the cervix occurs in virtually all women with first-attack genital herpes.

At the same time as the first symptoms appear, the skin becomes reddened and fluid-filled blisters (also called vesicles) appear on the external genitals. The commonest sites involved are the mons pubis, the labia majora, the labia minora, the clitoris, the fourchette and the vaginal introitus. The skin around the anus may also be involved. If the woman has had anal sex the anal canal may be infected (see anal herpes below). The blisters are usually painful and often surrounded by red painful skin. The number of blisters is variable, ranging from one or two up to several dozen. After a few days, the blisters burst to leave weeping painful sores. Sometimes the blisters burst very rapidly and may not even be recognised by the patient. In some patients the blisters (and subsequent ulcers) occur in crops, a few every two to three days for up to two weeks. After a further seven to ten days the ulcers on the skin (labia majora, perineum, mons and perianal area) form scabs or crusts which fall off to leave normal skin. The sores on the mucous membranes (the wet skin on the inner aspect of the labia minora, urethra, fourchette) heal without scabs or crusts. Healing is often accompanied by itching.

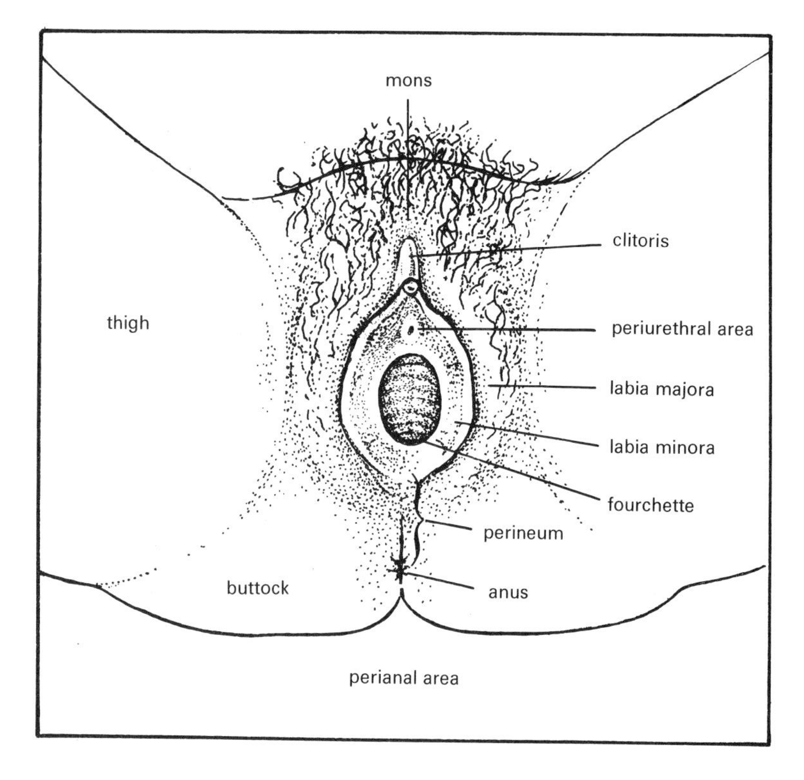

Commonly affected female genital areas in recurrent genital herpes.

The symptoms begin to improve after seven to ten days and the entire illness lasts anywhere from one to four weeks. However, some women feel tired and listless for several weeks after.

MEN

The infection can involve the penis or the perianal skin and the anal canal. Penile herpes is usually less severe than genital herpes in women; in contrast, perianal and anal herpes is usually a severe and prolonged illness.

Penile herpes

Although penile herpes is usually less severe than genital herpes in women, in most other respects the illnesses are similar. The first symptoms occur two to fourteen days following exposure and consist of pain and, in some patients, fever and flu-like symptoms. At the same time, painful fluid-filled blisters surrounded by red inflamed skin occur on the penis, the commonest sites involved being the glans, coronal sulcus, prepuce and shaft. If the sores are in or near the urethra (the tube from which the urine flows), pain on urination or a urethral discharge may occur. Sometimes blisters may be noticed on the scrotum or the groins. As in women, the blisters soon burst to leave painful weeping ulcers that eventually scab over and then heal. Painful swellings in the groin may be noticed due to inflammation of the lymph glands (see above). The entire illness lasts one to three weeks.

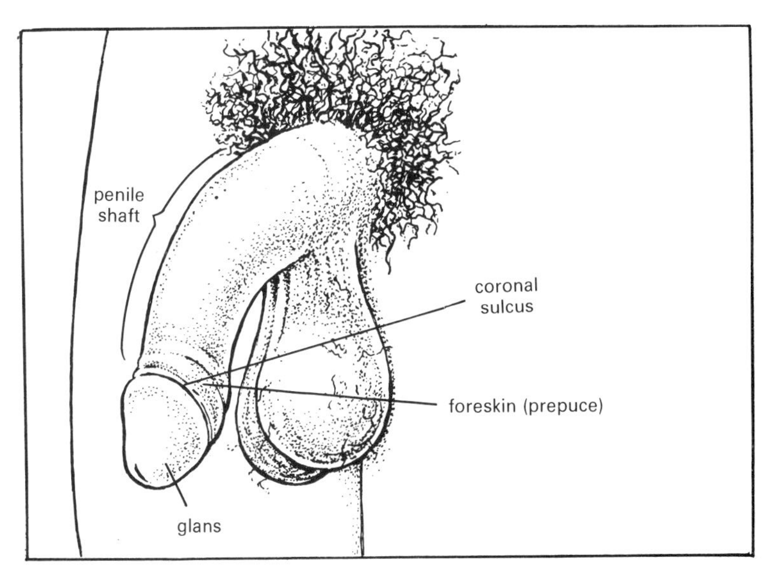

Commonly affected male genital areas in recurrent genital herpes.

Occasionally, the sores may occur only inside the urethra. When this happens the only symptoms are a discharge from the urethra and pain on urination. In this situation special tests (see below) are required to differentiate the infection from gonorrhoea and non-specific urethritis.

Perianal and anal herpes

In homosexual men who have had passive anal sex, or women who have had anal sex, herpes may occur on the perianal skin and inside the anus. The symptoms occur two to fourteen days after exposure, the first symptom being pain in or around the anus, often accompanied by an anal discharge, bleeding and pain on defaecation. The discharge and bleeding are due to infection within the anus. Fever and flu-like symptoms are common. Painful blisters and then weeping open sores are often noticed on the perianal skin. The lymph glands in the groin may be enlarged and painful. The pain associated with this condition is usually severe. The sores eventually heal; however, the illness is often prolonged, lasting anything up to four weeks, and feelings of general ill health and debility may last considerably longer.

RECURRENT GENITAL HERPES

Recurrences of genital herpes are usually less severe and of shorter duration than the first attack; most recurrences only last six or seven days, although occasionally they may be considerably longer.

The attacks often commence with warning or prodromal (preceding) symptoms, the nature of these symptoms being extremely variable. A common warning symptom is a burning or tingling sensation in the skin at the site where the blisters or ulcers subsequently occur. In some patients there may be pain or swelling of the lymph glands in the groin; some feel generally unwell, others have fevers or odd aches and pains. Many people develop neuralgia (nerve pain) in the groin, buttock, thigh, genital area, or down the back of the leg. These symptoms usually occur a few hours before the blisters appear, although in some people they occur several days before the disease manifests itself. It is not uncommon for the warning symptoms to occur with no subsequent blisters or sores. Many people find that the warning symptoms, especially the neuralgia pain, are the most troublesome aspect of the illness.

However, some people have no warning of an impending attack. The first they know of it is when they notice some pain or discomfort, and then recognise the typical blisters or sores. The neuralgia pain may, on occasion, occur at the same time as when the blisters first appear, rather than as a warning symptom.

The first sign of an outbreak is often slight redness of the skin, followed within a few hours by blisters. These burst to leave ulcers which heal by scabbing over. Frequently the redness and blisters are transient and not even noticed by the patient. Most recurrences occur on the external genitals: in women, the labia majora, labia minora, fourchette, perineum around the clitoris and the groin; in men, the penis and occasionally the groin or scrotum. Patients who have had previous perianal and anal herpes tend to have recurrences on the perianal skin. Internal lesions are very uncommon with recurrent genital herpes. There is usually only a simple or small group of blisters (and then ulcers) associated with each recurrence, but occasionally two or more recurrences at different anatomical sites may occur concurrently or sequentially. Recurrence on the thighs or buttocks are common, even in people who did not have this site involved with the first attack. This is because the nerves serving the thighs and buttocks are the same as those of the genitals, and when the virus reactivates in the nerve cells in the sacral ganglia (see Chapter 1) it can come down any of the branches of that nerve. The pain associated with each outbreak is usually mild and short lived; many people describe it as discomfort rather than pain. Sometimes there may be mild pain during or after urination, particularly if the ulcers are near the urethra. Fevers and flu-like symptoms are uncommon.

Women tend to have more in the way of symptoms than men, although on average men have slightly longer recurrences. The frequency and severity of recurrences is enormously variable, both from person to person and in the same person from one recurrence to the next. The average recurrence lasts six to seven days; however, recurrences as short as two days or as long as three weeks are not uncommon. Occasionally scars or marks may persist on the skin, particularly if recurrences occur repeatedly at the same site.

Abortive recurrences

Many people find that, on occasion, they develop the warning symptoms mentioned above, or even a bit of redness, but that no blisters or ulcers occur, and the entire episode is over in a few hours. These abortive episodes probably represent very transient recurrences. None the less, patients should regard themselves as being infectious at this time.

INAPPARENT HERPES

Occasionally people may attend their doctor for a routine check-up or a smear test, or because of some minor genital symptom, and the doctor or nurse may see a small ulcer which on culture (see below) turns out to be herpes. In these circumstances, on close questioning patients often reveal that they have had occasional pain or noticed small cuts or ulcers in the genital area which they thought were either of no significance, or which they attributed to recent sexual activity, masturbation or minor injury.

SEXUALLY TRANSMITTED ORAL HERPES

From time to time oral herpes may be contracted as a result of orogenital contact with somebody who had vulval or penile herpes. Patients complain of a sore throat and swollen painful glands in the neck, and the throat may look red and ulcerated on examination. The condition is often confused with other causes of a sore throat, including glandular fever and streptococcal sore throat.

The condition is self-limiting, resolving in 10–14 days. Often the possibility of herpes is not considered and the patient is treated with antibiotics for a bacterial sore throat. The condition may recur as cold sores on the lips.

Oral herpes (cold sores) and genital herpes

Cold sores are usually caused by *Herpes simplex* type 1, although infections with HSV 2 also occur. As with genital herpes, people with cold sores have recurrences. People with cold sores can transmit the infection to the genitals of their sexual partners during orogenital sex and, as mentioned above, people with genital herpes can transmit the infection to the mouth and lips of their sexual partners. Transfer from one person's mouth to their own genitals (or vice versa) via fingers does not appear to occur.

People who have previously had oral herpes are less likely to contract genital herpes as this earlier infection gives some degree of immune protection. If someone with previous oral herpes does get genital herpes the first episode is usually less severe, but the likelihood, frequency and severity of any subsequent recurrences is unaltered.

DIAGNOSING HERPES

The clinical features of first-attack genital herpes are often severe and are usually readily recognised by the doctor. As discussed above, recurrent outbreaks are usually less severe and the features may not be suggestive of herpes. But in most circumstances, even when herpes is obvious, the doctor will often wish to confirm the diagnosis by taking special tests; this may involve taking scrapings from blisters or sores, and may be quite painful.

Any person with sores on the genitals should seek medical advice as there are numerous causes for this complaint, although herpes is one of the commonest causes. However, other conditions, including various infections and skin conditions, may need to be excluded by the doctor; these include the following:

- Infections
  - Syphilis.
  - Tropical sexually transmitted infections – chancroid, lymphogranuloma venereum and granuloma inguinale.
  - Candida (thrush).
  - Trichomononiasis.
  - Scabies.
- Non-infectious causes
  - Trauma or injury.
  - Reiter's syndorme.
  - Behcet's syndrome.
  - Reaction to drugs.
  - Skin diseases.

In the Western world genital herpes is the commonest cause of genital ulceration, but in the tropics and subtropics chancroid and other tropical infections are more common. Chancroid is a bacterial infection that usually reveals itself two to five days after sexual exposure. Painful ulcers appear on the genitals, associated with enlarged and painful lymph glands in the groin. Unlike herpes, the condition does not usually resolve without treatment, but with antibiotics it is rapidly cured. It does not recur. The other tropical infections – lymphogranuloma venereum and granuloma inguinale – are far less common than chancroid and they are seldom confused with herpes.

Syphilis is a sexually transmitted disease caused by a bacterium called *Treponema pallidum.* The first sign of infection is an ulcer appearing on the genitals, mouth or anus three to six weeks after exposure. The ulcer is usually painless and single, although multiple and/or painful ulceration may occur. The lymph glands in the groin are often enlarged, but they are not usually tender. The condition can be readily diagnosed by means of taking special scrapings from the ulcer, and blood tests.

Thrush is a common fungal (yeast) infection, especially in women. It may cause a vaginal discharge and itching, and sometimes superficial sores on the vulva that may be confused with herpes. Trichomoniasis is also a common infection; it is caused by a parasite, and usually causes a vaginal discharge, soreness of the vulva and occasionally superficial sores on the vulva.

Scabies is an infection caused by a parasite called *Sarcoptes scabeii.* It is transmitted by close physical contact, and typically occurs in schoolchildren around the hands and arms. However it sometimes occurs in adults in the genital area. The parasite burrows under the skin, and these burrows may occasionally be confused with herpes.

Injury to the vulva or penis, for example from over-vigorous sex, reaction to various drugs, and a number of skin disorders, can all sometimes be confused with herpes.

Reiter's syndrome is a rare disease usually affecting men. Problems include a urethral discharge, ulcers on the glans penis, swollen joints, sore eyes and various skin rashes. The ulcers on the penis may on occasion cause confusion with herpes. The cause of Reiter's syndrome is unknown; however, it is known to occur as a consequence of various bowel or genital infections.

Behcet's syndrome is an extremely rare disease, of unknown cause. Problems include swollen joints, rashes, brain problems and recurrent painful ulcers of the mouth and genitals, and may rarely be confused with herpes.

LABORATORY DIAGNOSIS OF HERPES

There are a number of methods of diagnosing herpes in the laboratory. The most common, reliable and widely used is a technique called cell culture. This involves transporting a scraping from the blisters or sores to the laboratory in a glass or plastic tube containing special chemicals and nutrients which are able to keep the virus alive. On arrival a small portion of the specimen is placed in containers housing living cells that have been grown in the laboratory. The virus is able to multiply in these cells, and within a few days changes occur in the cells

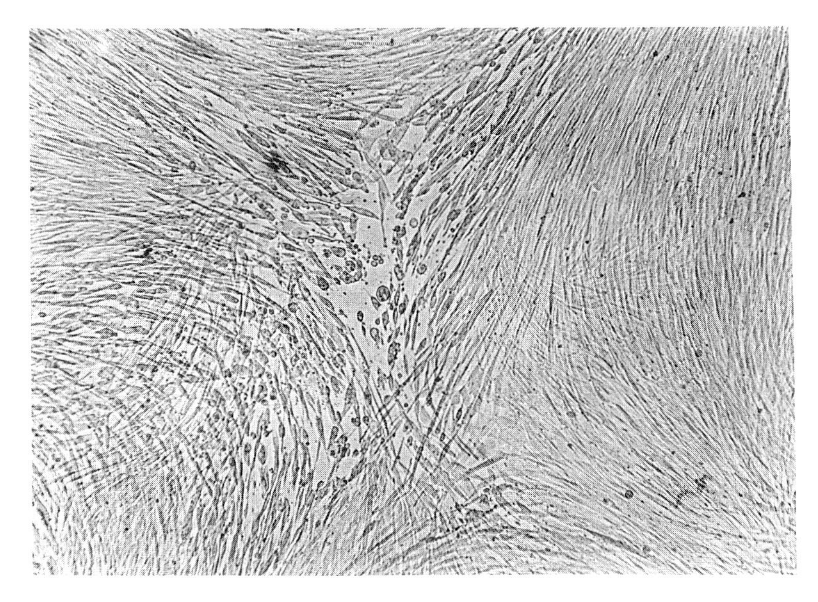

(a)

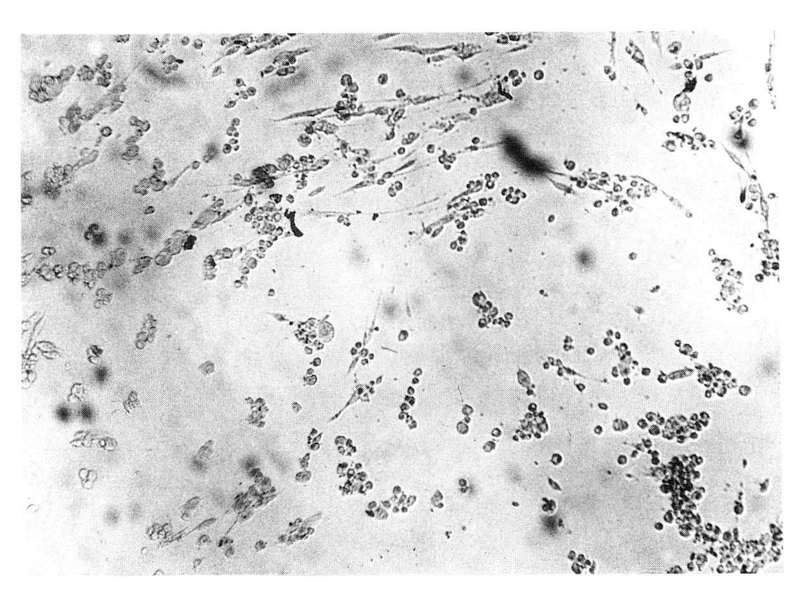

(b)

Effect of herpes on laboratory cell cultures, as seen under the microscope. In (a) the cells are rounding up — an early sign of damage — while in (b) there are no live cells.

which may be readily identified under the microscope as typical of herpes infection. Whilst this method is the 'gold standard', it has the disadvantage of taking from two to seven days to get an answer.

There are a number of other methods available for identifying herpes; many of these are rapid, but none are as accurate as the culture technique mentioned above. One simple method is to obtain material from scraping a blister or sore, putting it on to a microscope slide, staining it with special stains and examining it under a microscope. Cells infected with herpes show changes in the nucleus (called intranuclear inclusions) which are only seen with herpes virus infections. Unfortunately, this simple test shows up the infection only in a small percentage of patients. Occasionally, when a cervical smear (cancer or Pap smear) is taken from a woman who has active herpes of the cervix, similar changes may be seen.

There are several tests available which rely on the detection of herpes antigens from specimens (antigens being those parts of the virus which are able to stimulate the immune system). The sophistication and accuracy of these tests have increased enormously over recent years and some of the tests currently available are almost as reliable as cell culture. All these tests give a rapid answer (the result is usually available in two to three hours), and some have the added advantage of telling whether the infection is due to HSV 1 or HSV 2.

All the tests mentioned above depend upon the presences of active herpes, i.e. the presence of blisters or sores. But one of the most difficult problems is to confirm the diagnosis of herpes in someone who only has very infrequent recurrences, or in contacts who give no history of previous herpes infection (see Chapter 1). Unfortunately, at present, there is no test which can help in this situation.

It is sometimes suggested that blood tests may help as antibodies to *Herpes simplex* (see Chapter 1) can be detected in the blood. But unfortunately the information derived from these tests is limited; until very recently, most blood tests could not differentiate accurately between antibodies to HSV 1 and HSV 2. Consequently, as a considerable percentage of the adult population have previously been exposed to herpes (usually oral HSV 1 – see Chapter 1), the presence of antibodies merely indicates that the individual has at some time been exposed to the virus; it does not tell us if the infection is oral or genital herpes (or indeed both), nor if the condition is currently active, nor if the individual is infectious. Whilst these blood tests are sometimes used to reassure people or as 'evidence' of genital

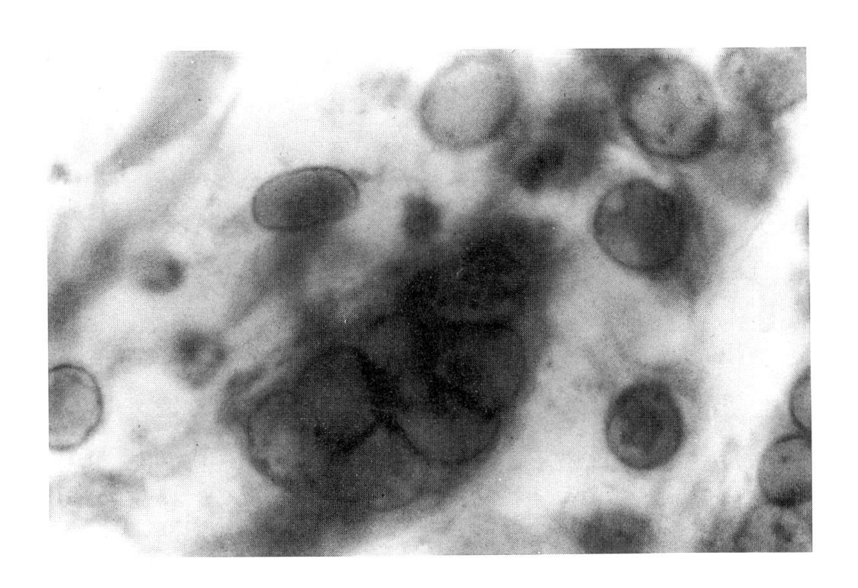

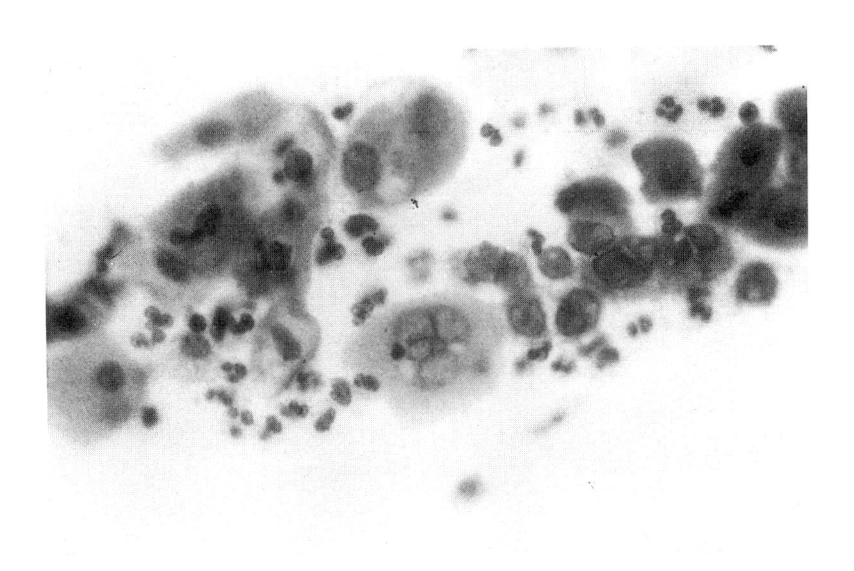

Cells, obtained by scraping a blister or sore, infected with herpes.

herpes, our own view is that they are of no value and should not be offered to people.

Recently, workers in America have developed antibody blood tests which reliably differentiate between HSV 1 and HSV 2. These tests are vastly superior to the other antibody tests, but still do not tell if the infection is oral or genital, or if it is active. However these tests are proving very valuable in studies of the epidemiology, transmission and clinical features of herpes.

OTHER CONDITIONS CAUSED BY HERPES

Infection with HSV may cause a variety of clinical problems other than genital herpes. It should be stressed that these are not associated with genital herpes; they are other types of infection that may occur with HSV.

Cold sores (oral herpes)

Herpes infections of the lips and mouth are very common. They are usually acquired in childhood and, like genital herpes, may recur from time to time. As with genital herpes, the virus remains in a latent or inactive state between recurrences, the site of latency being a group of nerve cells near the ear called the trigeminal ganglion. As discussed above, oral herpes may be spread to the genitalia, and vice versa.

Eye infection

HSV may infect the eyes. This usually occurs as a result of direct introduction of the virus into the eye or, very occasionally, as a consequence of reactivation of latent virus from the trigeminal ganglion (see above).

Herpes eye infection is usually very painful and if left untreated may damage the eye and lead to loss of vision. Infection is mostly confined to the surface of the eye, but involvement of the deeper structures can occur. Early treatment with antiviral drugs is very successful. It should be stressed that oral herpes is common, but eye infection is rare.

Widespread skin disease

Herpes is known to complicate several skin diseases, the commonest being eczema. This usually occurs in children who present to the doctor with widespread eczema and herpes over much of the body. Some children may be extremely ill, with high fevers and the possibility of spread of the infection to internal organs. Antiviral drugs, in particular acyclovir (see Chapter 5), may be life saving in these circumstances.

Herpes of the internal organs

In patients whose immune system is not working efficiently HSV may very rarely spread to various internal organs, including the liver, lungs and the oesophagus (gullet). This is also an extremely serious situation and treatment with acyclovir may again be very helpful (see Chapter 5).

Herpes encephalitis

Encephalitis (inflammation of the brain) is the most feared problem caused by HSV. It is difficult to recognise, and diagnosis and treatment is often unsatisfactory. How the virus reaches the brain is the subject of considerable debate and controversy. Fortunately encephalitis is exceptionally rare.

3

PROBLEMS

There are a number of complications and long-term consequences that may occur in association with genital herpes. Some occur with the first attack, and usually cause no subsequent problem; these include urinary difficulties, meningitis and a condition called sacral radiculomyelopthy. These will be discussed in detail below. Several other issues that will be considered in this chapter include the spread of herpes to sites distant from the genitalia, herpes in pregnancy, and the possible association of genital herpes with cervical cancer.

URINARY PROBLEMS

Difficulty with urination, or even complete inability to urinate, are not at all uncommon in patients with a first attack of genital herpes. This is due to blisters or ulcers near or actually inside the urethra. When the person urinates the urine touches the open sores and causes severe pain, a situation particularly common in women, where the sores are often on the inner aspect of the labia minora and around the urethra. The pain may be so severe that the person may be totally unable to pass urine, a condition called urinary retention. Sometimes this persists even when the sores are getting better because of the fear and anxiety associated with the earlier pain.

SACRAL RADICULOMYELOPATHY

Urinary problems may also be associated with a neurological problem called sacral radioculomyelopathy, in which the herpes infection may affect the nerve cells at the base of the spine (see illustration on page 5). This condition occurs commonly in men with perianal and anal herpes, and very occasionally in women with vulval or men with penile herpes. The condition only occurs with primary infections, and has never been described with recurrences. Although this problem usually occurs when the patient has a very severe primary infection, it can also occur with less severe infections.

Patients with this complaint develop problems with urination and defaecation, pain in the back of the thigh or buttocks, decreased skin sensitivity around the anal or genital area and, in men, problems obtaining an erection. It usually lasts two to three weeks, gets better spontaneously and does not cause any long-term neurological problems.

The management both of urinary problems and of sacral radiculomyelopathy is discussed in Chapter 5.

MENINGITIS

Meningitis is a condition caused by inflammation of the membranes (called meninges) that surround the brain. There

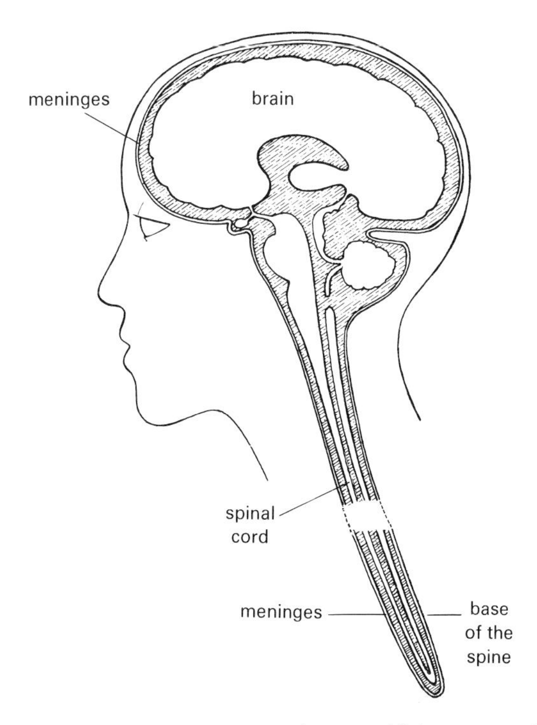

The herpes virus can infect the meninges which surround the brain and spinal cord.

are a large number of bacteria and viruses that can cause meningitis, and herpes is one of them. The meningitis associated with some infections may be very serious; however, with *Herpes simplex* the infection is mild, short lived, recovers completely within a few days, and there are no long-term neurological consequences.

Herpes meningitis usually occurs if the patient has a severe primary genital infection. Fever and headache are early symptoms. The headache may get progressively worse and after a few days there may be intolerance to bright light (a condition called photophobia) and stiffness of the neck. On very rare occasions the doctor may be so concerned about the condition that admission to hospital is recommended. A lumbar puncture – draining off a small quantity of the cerebrospinal fluid which surrounds the brain and spinal cord by inserting a small needle between the bones of the spine – may be performed to confirm the diagnosis.

The management of this condition is discussed in Chapter 6.

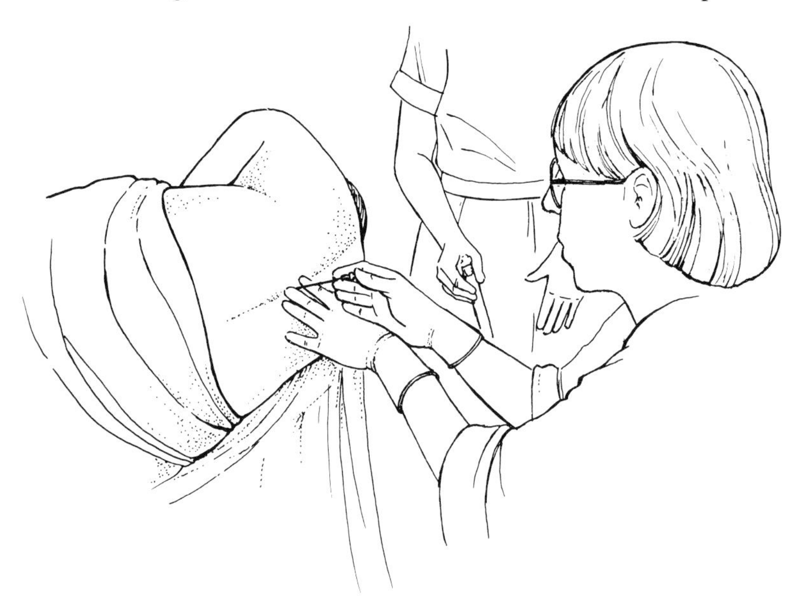

Lumber puncture being performed.

SPREAD OF HERPES ON THE BODY

Blisters and/or ulcers associated with genital herpes may occur anywhere on the body; they may be associated with the first attack and may subsequently recur at the same or adjacent skin

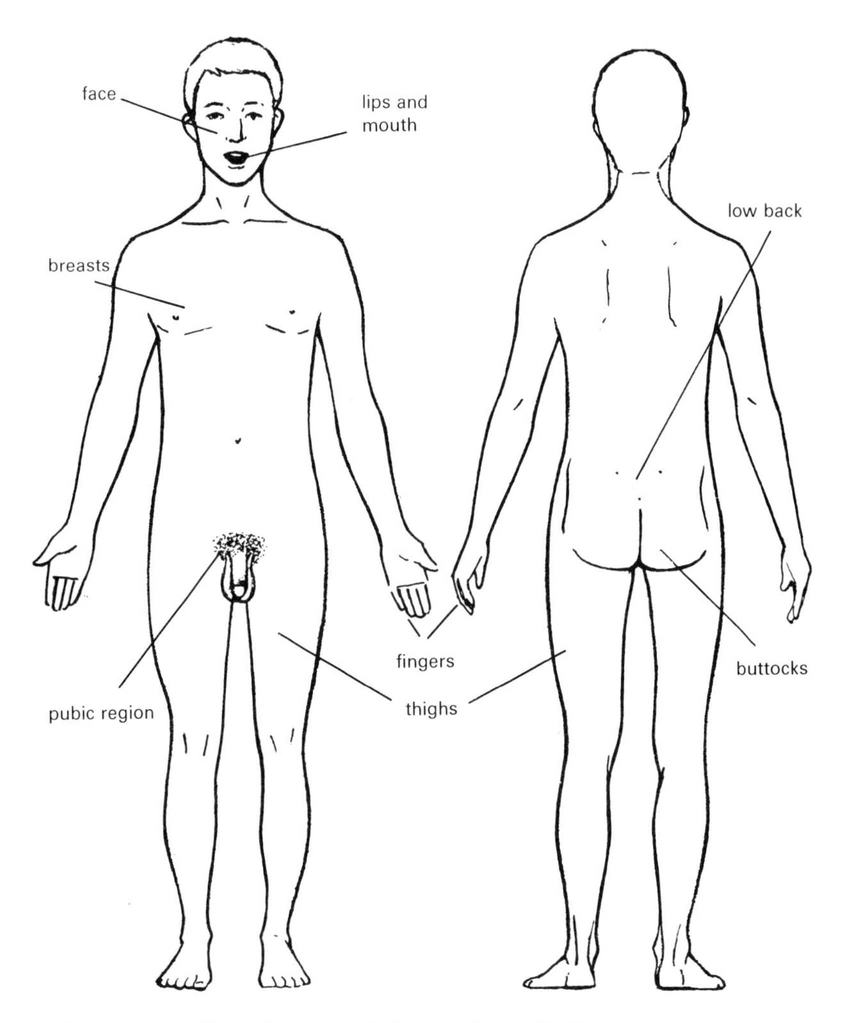

Commonly affected non-genital areas in genital herpes.

sites. The commonest sites involved are on the hands, fingers, thighs, lips, mouth, face, buttocks and breasts.

It is probable that such blisters/ulcers occur as a consequence of direct inoculation at that site during sexual activity at the time when the infection is first contracted, although some people believe that they occur by spread through the blood, or by transfer from one skin site to another (this last explanation seems unlikely as one would then expect to see infection of the hands and fingers far more frequently). In some people several different sites may be involved.

The blisters and ulcers are very similar to those occurring on the genitals. They may be very painful and, in areas where the skin is thick, may last several weeks. In some people the infection may recur at these skin sites, but not on the genitals; in others they may occur on the hands, face or other skin sites only with the first attack and then, even if the person has frequent genital recurrences, no further skin outbreaks occur. In contrast, patients who only have genital recurrences sometimes suddenly develop blisters or sores on the thighs or buttocks. It is believed that this occurs because the nerves serving the genital area are the same as those serving the thighs and buttocks and the virus, instead of coming down the same branches of the nerve, come down an adjacent branch (see Chapter 2).

Skin blisters or sores are infectious and herpes can be transmitted if these come into contact with a susceptible individual.

HERPES IN PREGNANCY AND NEWBORN BABIES

Genital herpes may be spread to the newborn baby via the mother's birth canal (cervix, vagina and vulva) if the mother has herpes at the time. Infection in newborns is extremely uncommon, but when it does occur it can be a very serious infection.

In some babies the infection only involves the skin, mouth or eyes, and usually resolves with no long-term consequences. More commonly the infection involves the brain, lungs and other internal organs; this is a very serious situation, with many of these babies dying and a considerable number of the survivors having serious brain damage.

The risk of spread from mother to baby depends upon several factors. The greatest risk to the baby is when the mother is having a first attack of genital herpes at or around the onset of labour. This is because first-attack genital herpes is usually severe, with the cervix and vulva often involved and considerable quantities of infectious virus present. In addition, because the mother has not yet produced protective antibodies, none are available to be transferred via the placenta to the baby. (Maternal antibodies are transfered across the placenta and protect the baby against infection during the first few months of life before it has an opportunity to develop its own antibodies.)

The risk of spread to the newborn from a mother who has recurrent genital herpes is very much less. This is because most recurrences involve the vulva and not the cervix; during delivery the newborn is often in prolonged contact with the cervix, whereas contact with the vulva is usually short lived. Furthermore, the amount of virus present is usually small, and the baby often has protective antibodies from the mother.

The management of herpes in pregnancy is discussed in Chapter 5.

GENITAL HERPES AND CERVICAL CARCINOMA

Cervical cancer is one of the commonest cancers to affect women. The exact cause (or causes) of cervical cancer remain unknown, but a number of factors are now known to be associated. Many of these factors are related to the women's sexual activity, and include the following:

- Early age at first sexual intercourse.
- Greater number of sexual partners.
- Early age of marriage.
- Multiple marriages.

In addition to the sexual activity of the women, the sexual habits of her partner or partners are also known to be important. In some communities men often frequent prostitutes, whilst the women usually remain faithful to their partners; this occurs commonly in several South American countries, and in these communities cervical cancer is common. Additional evidence of the 'male factor' comes from several studies that have shown that the subsequent sexual partners of men whose first wives died because of cervical cancer were at a greatly increased risk of themselves developing cervical cancer. Finally, it is also known that the sexual contacts of men with penile cancer often have cervical cancer.

All of this evidence points to an agent or agents involved in cervical cancer that may be sexually transmitted, and over the years several sexually transmissable diseases have been considered, amongst them the following:

- *Chlamydia trachomatis*, a bacterial infection which is the cause of non-specific genital infection in men and infection of the cervix in women.
- *Trichomonas vaginalis*, a common sexually transmitted parasitic infection often causing a frothy offensive vaginal discharge.

- Syphilis.
- Cytomegalovirus, a virus similar to *Herpes simplex*, usually causing no symptoms (see Chapter 1).
- *Herpes simplex* itself.
- Human papilloma virus, the cause of genital warts.

Most authorities have dismissed all but the last two as being possibly associated with cervical cancer.

The cervix and cancer

Before considering the evidence suggesting a possible link between HSV and cervical cancer, it is helpful to consider the changes that can occur in the cervix before and during the development of cancer.

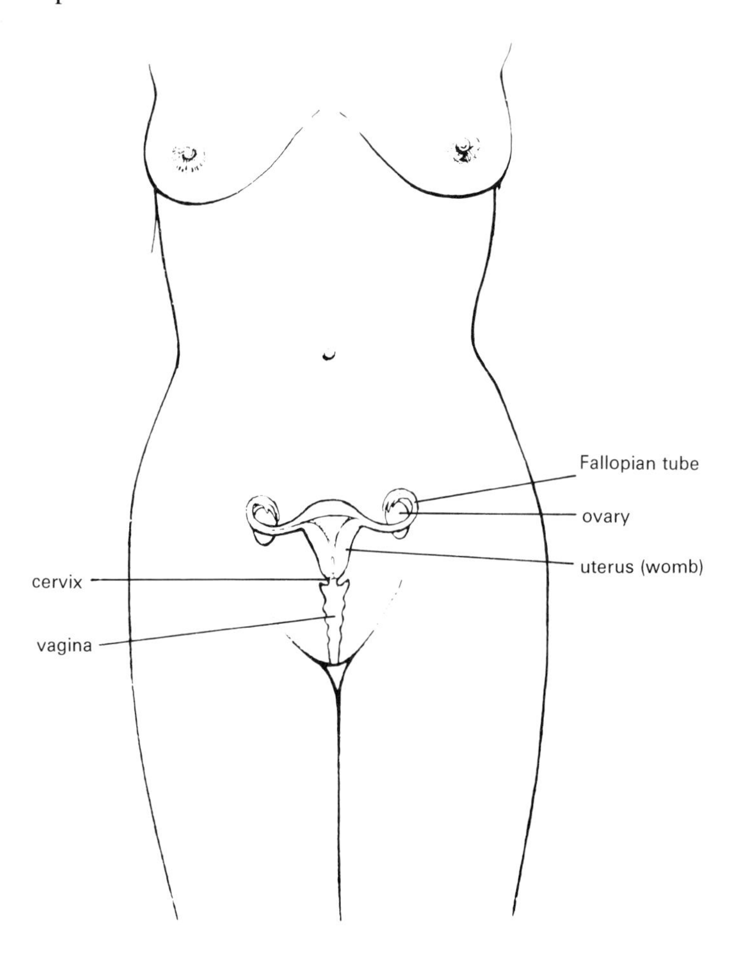

Position of the cervix.

The cervix is the lower part of the uterus (womb), linking the vagina with the womb. The cervix has a hole in it through which sperm can pass to fertilise the ovum (egg) and out of which the menstrual blood can come, and this hole stretches during labour to allow the birth of the baby. The outer part of the cervix is lined with tough cells called squamous epithelium, while the inner aspect is lined with a thin lining called the columnar epithelium. The two linings link up near the cervical hole, and this area is called the squamocolumnar junction; at this site the columnar cells slowly change to squamous cells, a normal process called squamous metaplasia. It is cells from this area that are examined microscopically after a cervical smear test.

It is these changing cells that potentially change into the wrong kind of cells and in some circumstances ultimately

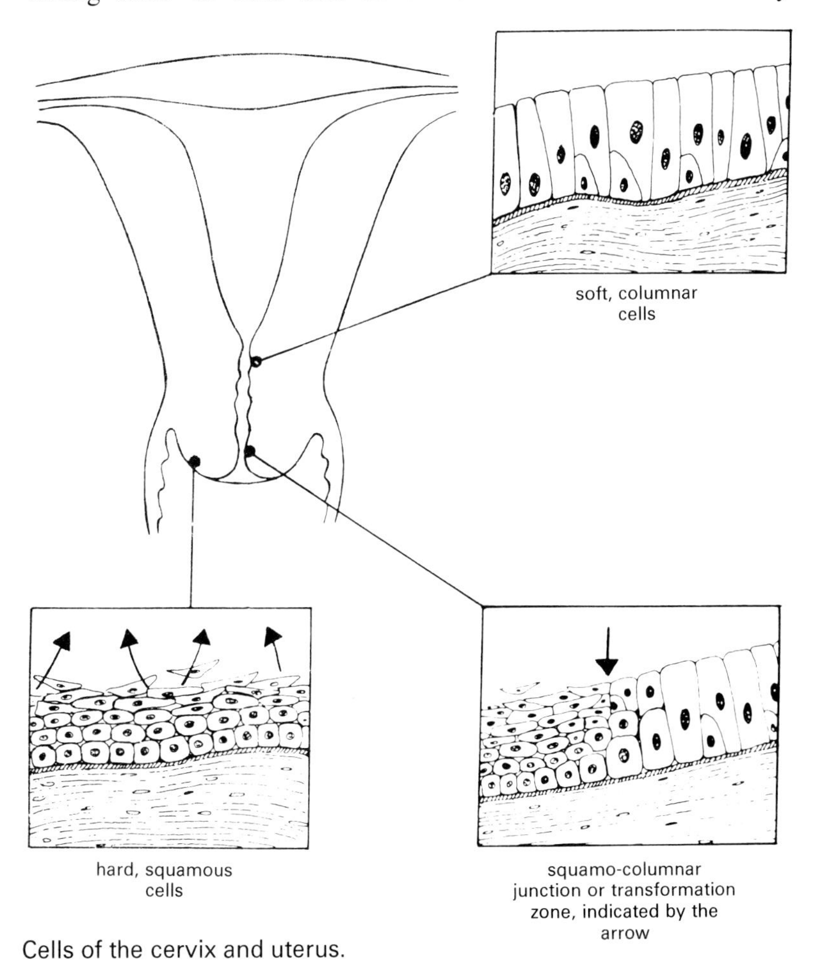

Cells of the cervix and uterus.

become cancer cells. These early changes can be recognised microscopically and are either called:

- Dysplasia – mild, moderate or severe.
- Or cervical intraepithelial neoplasia (CIN), graded as CIN I, II or III, corresponding to mild, moderate or severe dysplasia.

Many of these changes revert back to normal, although the more advanced the changes are (especially CIN III) the less likely this is to occur.

The evidence suggesting a possible link between *Herpes simplex* and cervical cancer may be considered under two headings, epidemiology and virology.

Epidemiological evidence

In the 1960s and early 1970s a number of studies were conducted in many different parts of the world to see if patients with cancer had antibodies to herpes in their blood. These studies showed that herpes antibodies were present in the majority of patients with cervical cancer, in a smaller percentage in the group that showed the early changes on the smear test (CIN), and in a still smaller proportion of the women with normal cervices. The conclusion reached was that, as the incidence of herpes antibodies was high in the group of women that also showed a high incidence of cervical cancer, the herpes was therefore a likely causative agent of the cancer.

However, the results of these studies have been criticised for several reasons. Firstly, as mentioned in Chapter 2, the blood tests used to detect HSV antibodies are unreliable and often will not differentiate adequately between HSV 1 and HSV 2. What this means is that these tests give a false impression of the number of infections due to genital herpes, as many of the positive results could be due to previous oral herpes (cold sores). A second reason is that many of the studies did not ascertain very reliable sexual histories from participating women, and it has been suggested that the presence of herpes antibodies may only indicate more sexual activity. In other words the more sexual intercourse a woman has with different partners, the more likely she is to come into contact with herpes and also the more likely she is to develop cervical cancer, i.e. the two factors (herpes and cervical cancer) are perhaps only linked in an independent way.

The results of studies with the newer types of specific antibody tests are awaited with interest and may help to unravel this complex issue.

The virological evidence

There are several indirect strands of virological evidence which point towards a possible link between HSV and cervical cancer. Firstly, a number of animal viruses belonging to the herpes group have been implicated in the causation of several tumours in a variety of animals, including chickens, frogs and monkeys. In addition, in man there is evidence linking two rare tumours called Burkitt's lymphoma (a tumour of the lymph glands) and nasopharyngeal carcinoma (cancer of the upper throat) with a human herpes virus called Epstein-Barr virus (see Chapter 1).

The direct evidence consists, firstly, of the observation that *Herpes simplex* can alter certain cells grown in the laboratory, making them more likely to develop the changes associated with early cancer. Secondly, numerous experiments have been conducted looking for evidence of HSV DNA (the genetic material at the core of the virus) or HSV antigens – both telltale traces of herpes – in material taken from cervical cancer. There is no convincing evidence that HSV DNA can be found in cervical cancer, but herpes antigens have been reported by some scientists, although here too the evidence is far from convincing.

In recent years attention has shifted to another virus, the human papilloma virus (HPV, the cause of genital warts) as a more likely candidate to be associated with cervical carcinoma. But many workers still believe that additional factors (usually called cofactors) may be required, and it is possible that herpes may be just such a cofactor; other possible cofactors include smoking and other sexually transmitted diseases. The two theories (HSV as a primary cause of cervical cancer, and HSV as a cofactor) are summarised in the diagram overleaf.

In practical terms what does all this mean? Most importantly it means that there is no proven link between herpes and cervical cancer. However, whilst there is still some doubt, we would suggest that women with a history of genital herpes should have a cervical smear taken every year. This will enable the doctor to detect any of the early precancerous changes to the cells of the cervix and to initiate treatment before cancer develops.

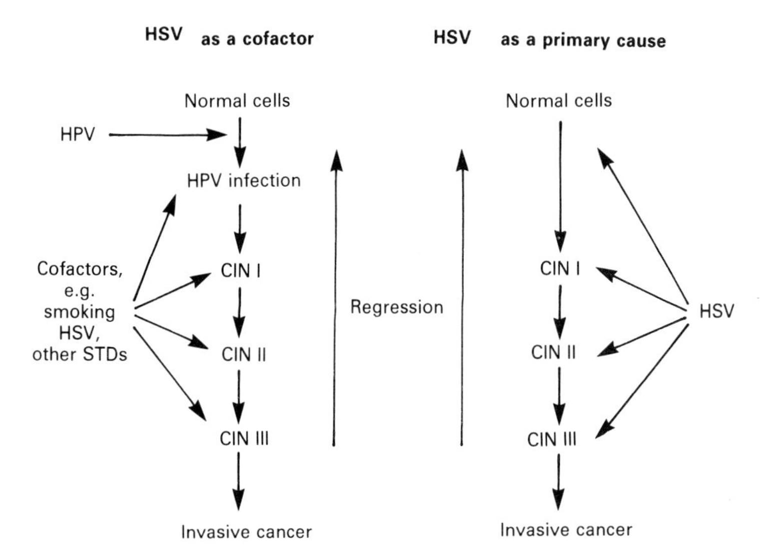

HPV = human papillomavirus (wart virus)
HSV = *Herpes simplex*
CIN = cervical intraepithelial neoplasia
STD = sexually transmitted disease

Two possible mechanisms underlying cervical cancer, *Herpes simplex* virus as a co-factor and *Herpes simplex* as a primary cause.

4

THE PSYCHOLOGY OF HERPES

When you're told that you have herpes, it's not uncommon to experience a whole myriad of emotions – from panic at one's lack of knowledge, to despair and anger at contracting it. This chapter will discuss not only these emotions, and the most common areas of anxiety for people with herpes – transmission of the disease, and how to tell partners – but also what to do and where to go if you want information, help and support.

In the early 1980s herpes received a lot of attention from the popular press and media, much of which was distorted and harmful. Thankfully, with the advent of HIV and AIDS, this attention has mostly stopped, but unfortunately the very real anxieties such attention engendered persist; because herpes is no longer in the news no one talks about it, and because no one talks about it ignorance about the virus persists.

Physically, for the majority of people with the infection, genital herpes is an occasionally recurrent, sometimes painful, skin condition. Some people do have very frequent or painful recurrences; for some it is the severe neuralgia prior to the recurrence which is so debilitating. For both groups it is the physical manifestations of the virus which are a problem, and long-term antiviral therapy can be of enormous benefit to them (see Chapter 5).

EMOTIONAL PROBLEMS

However, many people, regardless of the frequency or infrequency of attacks, find it hard to deal with the emotional aspect of the infection.

Herpes differs from the bacterial sexually transmitted infections like gonorrhoea because, although you can treat an outbreak, you cannot rid your body of the virus – it remains latent in the nerve ganglia. Conversely, herpes has no long-term debilitating effects on your physical health: gonorrhoea, if untreated however, can have serious implications, especially regarding women's fertility. Yet the word herpes carries emotive connotations which far outweigh its physical consequences; this is partly as already mentioned, a leftover from the pre-HIV era; but even with the subsequent health education and publicity given to sex and sexual practices, such matters are still treated with a mixture of coyness and salacious curiosity.

If it's the first time you have had herpes, or the first time you have been told that's what your symptoms have been, it's not unusual to feel incredulity, shock and panic – 'No, it can't be.' 'How on earth can I have got that?' 'I've had the same partner for three years, she/he must have been sleeping around.' Disbelief mingled with terrible anxiety can engulf people when they're told that they have herpes, because the only 'facts' they 'know' about the virus are that it's painful, it's incurable, and they can never have a sex life after this. And because of the shock, they don't absorb the correct information and advice.

If, when you leave the clinic, you can't remember anything you've been told, don't worry – make another appointment to see the doctor, nurse or health adviser. It's always wiser to ask rather than to speculate or to rely on what your friends tell you. It is understandable that some people shy away from asking for advice or returning to the clinic, but it must be emphasised that your queries and anxieties will be treated intelligently and sensitively.

However, it would be useful to discuss some of the emotions and difficulties some people have with herpes. Many of these relate to how sex and sexuality are still viewed. Bear in mind that sexually transmitted infections are still perceived as, on the one hand wilfully inflicted on 'innocent' parties, and, on the other, as just punishment for transgressing some 'moral code'.

With gonorrhoea – a bacterial infection – you can take your course of antibiotics and forget/pretend/deny that you ever had it. But viral infections like herpes (and warts) cannot be cured; they can only be treated, and the recurrences are often seen as a constant reminder of one's supposed promiscuity, infidelity, bad luck, victimisation.

It's not uncommon for people with herpes to put themselves in the role of innocent victim – 'I'm not a promiscuous person', the inference being that there are some others who have herpes for whom the virus is their just desserts. Or they feel that they were deliberately defiled, that the other person must have known that they had herpes. Or, one step further, they deny that they acquired it sexually at all, they were passive victims of infection from bedclothes, toilet seat, towels – again the suggestion that some people have herpes because they're 'promiscuous', whereas the individual in question is innocent and their behaviour was not culpable.

Conversely, some people view herpes as a punishment for some moral crime, that responding to your sexual needs and sexuality is something of which to be ashamed. You may feel guilty due to the circumstances by which you contracted herpes – extra-marital/relationship sex, sex when you are experimenting with your own sexuality. However, it's not uncommon to feel guilty for some unspecifiable reason and, because of this shame, you hide away, don't seek advice or information; you feel you should suffer in silence because you will be judged as guilty for your actions. What this does is perpetuate the notion (and reality) that herpes is something not talked about; you can't even tell your best friend, while at the same time you have to endure crass jokes about the virus.

Often connected with feelings of guilt and blame is the perception of actual physical stigma; the recurrences themselves are a constant reminder of your 'crime', that you are contaminated and dirty. For some this is an emotional response; for others the reaction is more physical, in that they are constantly trying to 'keep clean', ranging from zealous bathing to cleanliness in the moral sense – no more sexual activity because they feel that they are soiled or damaged goods.

Related to this attitude is the perception that the individual is contagious at all times, not only when they have an outbreak; that they are reservoirs of disease over which they have no control. This can spill over into everyday life – the unfounded fear that someone will catch herpes from using their cups, towels, bath, and in so doing will expose them as a carrier of the disease.

Because there is no set pattern, no rules as to what may happen when you have herpes, it is very easy to feel that your body is out of your control, that the virus holds you hostage to its capricious nature. You can't formulate new relationships or expand on existing ones because you never know what's going to happen, when the next sore is going to appear. For some it is not the actual outbreaks which upset them, as this is a physical reality which they control; instead it is the mental distress of anticipating when the next episode is going to come that severely limits their sexual and social lives. There is a feeling of 'Why bother?', because as soon as you meet someone, you're bound to get an attack, you won't be able to have sex with them, and you'll have to explain why.

Of course, not everyone who has herpes experiences these feelings, and for many who do they are fleeting. However, it's worth knowing that, although they are unique to the individual, other people have gone through the same demoralisation. Just as it's not shameful to have herpes, neither should you be ashamed of your feelings about the virus.

DEALING WITH THE PROBLEMS

Acknowledging these feelings is one thing, but how do you tackle them?

Firstly access to the correct information is vital in understanding herpes, thus allowing you to dispel some myths and fears; often anxieties are based on misinterpreted facts and erroneous advice. As already mentioned, if you're unsure about something, always ask; often repeated advice is preferable to solitary panicking. Once you've got the facts straight, you can look at how you perceive herpes. What do you feel, and why? For example:

- How do you describe herpes? In a roundabout fashion – 'My problem'? Euphemistically – 'The spot'? Emotionally – 'Dirty, ashamed, unclean'?
- When you have an outbreak, how do you feel mentally? Does it differ from when you don't have an outbreak, or does the very fact that you have herpes pervade your everyday life?
- Do you find yourself putting restrictions on what you can and can't do – for example, not going swimming when you have an attack in case someone sees it, or somehow contracts herpes from you in the pool?

Perceptions of, and anxieties about, herpes can be highlighted in the areas of transmission and telling partners.

Transmission

Fear of transmission is common. However, the only restriction herpes should have on your life, apart from if it's physically debilitating, is when you have sex – and this is only in its narrowest definition. From when/if you experience warning symptoms, e.g. tingling, pain in the buttocks or thighs, until the sore has healed, you should avoid close sexual contact with someone who doesn't have herpes.

The only way genital herpes is transmitted is from:

- Genital-to-genital contact.
- Mouth-to-genital contact.

In order to contract herpes, you have to have close skin-to-skin contact with someone who is shedding virus at that time, and from that specific part of the body where the skin-to-skin contact is occurring.

You don't need to have penetrative sex to acquire or transmit the virus, but it is the commonest mode because of the friction involved; the skin around the genitals is friable and only needs the tiniest abrasion for the virus to enter the skin (see Chapter 1). The same is true if you have oral sex with someone who has a cold sore around their mouth. Thus it is not a socially transmitted infection – you're not going to give someone herpes if you sit next to them, shake hands, share cups, cutlery, towels, toilet seats, bath water.

By knowing how herpes is transmitted you can minimise its interference in daily life. The restrictions on your sex life depend very much on the frequency of outbreaks, but despite this, it's important to remember that it's only close skin-to-skin contact with the part of the body where you get attacks which you should avoid; it does not mean that during an attack you can't cuddle, share beds, kiss (if you have no cold sores).

It's understandable that people are concerned about giving someone else herpes, but if you become aware of when you're having a recurrence, avoid close sexual contact when you do, and use condoms at other times, then this reduces the risk substantially (condom use and safer sex are discussed in Chapter 6).

Telling partners

Telling your partner you have herpes also removes a large area of anxiety. But this may not be as easy as it sounds: for some the fear of rejection, and of betrayal, is very real; for others this fear lies in unfounded assumptions, in that you imagine you know how other people would react to being told about herpes.

What you know and feel about herpes will be all too apparent in how you tell your partner – the medium really is as important as the message. Don't use euphemisms – tell the other person that you have herpes. If you tell someone that you have 'a problem that recurs every few months', it is unlikely that they will understand what you are talking about. So be honest and tell them exactly what it is and how it affects sexual relationships. Tell them:

- What herpes is.
- How it is transmitted.
- How often you have outbreaks.
- What you do when you have an outbreak.
- What you do to lessen the likelihood that they will contract herpes.

If there is a friend who knows you have herpes, try a 'dummy run' on them if you are anxious about how it will come across. If you sound as if herpes is something to be alarmed about, then your tone will be what the other person will pick up on, not how much you know about herpes.

- Don't tell a partner when you're drunk or stoned; you may feel you need Dutch courage, but it's not fair on the other person. And anyway you may not remember afterwards what you have said.
- Tell your partner as early on in the relationship as possible. Trust works both ways in a relationship, or prospective relationship, so that deciding when you tell someone means weighing up the need for honesty with another person against the risk that you might be endowing the relationship with a greater degree of intimacy than either of you are prepared for – you may well not wish to tell someone you have just met something which you find embarrassing or painful. However if you've had sex with someone whom you have not told, it's then very easy to speculate – What if? What happens when?

So why do some people not tell their partners that they have herpes?

- Fear of rejection.
- Fear of false assumptions about their past behaviour.
- Fear of gossip.
- Fear their partner won't understand.

The only way to overcome those fears is to tell someone and to be sure of your facts. But it is also important to ask yourself 'Why should that other person walk off if I tell them that I have herpes?' 'Why should they gossip about something I've told them in confidence?' 'Why do I think that's how they will react?' Again, your answers are based on your assumptions, in which you transfer your anxieties on to someone else. It's no good just saying to yourself that 'Anyone would run a mile if I told them I've got herpes', when what you mean is that you're still coming to terms with it in your own mind and would find it difficult to present the idea of herpes in anything less than a lurid and distressing way.

It's true that when you're feeling anxious and demoralised about something, it's often difficult to put it into perspective. But the majority of people aren't going to be alarmed or discouraged by the fact that you have herpes, and the personal satisfaction and relief of sharing your worries with another person can be enormous; the more people you tell – friends, family, lovers, etc. – the less of a mystique and big deal it becomes.

And what happens if those fears do become a reality?

- Rejection can be very painful and distressing and make you even more loath to tell anyone else that you have herpes. But you must challenge the person who's rejecting you and ask them why? What is it that they can't/won't accept? If you've told them what herpes is, how it's transmitted, what you do to reduce the risk of transmission – that is, if you have been straight and honest with them – and they won't accept this, perhaps they're using herpes as a convenient (and sometimes smugly self-righteous) excuse to terminate the relationship.
- They make assumptions about you – that you've been sleeping around, you're promiscuous. It's a popular and hypocritical myth that 'nice' people don't get sexually transmitted infections. But anyone who is sexually active is at risk of acquiring such infections. If others want to make snide allusions to your supposed past, leave them to it – don't go on the defensive. You've got nothing to be ashamed of.
- Gossip. It's understandable that, because you're worried about something, you feel it's beyond your control, and so you imagine that it will be literally beyond your control – that people will start talking about you if you tell someone. Undoubtedly there are those who are so shallow that the sexual lives of other people are the greatest source of their conversation. But would your partner, lover, best friend really use your intimate concerns as fuel for juicy gossip?

- Sex and sexuality bring out the inarticulate and euphemistic in all of us. It can be difficult enough to discuss desires and wants within sexual relationships without having to explain what herpes is. But, as has already been said what you need to know is what herpes is, how it affects you and your partner and what is involved on the emotional side. If your partner looks blank, alarmed, puzzled, ask them if they understand what you're telling them, and if they don't, go through it again.

And what happens if they do get herpes? Perhaps you think that could be the worst thing you could do to someone else? But why? You're the one who has it, you know what it's like physically and mentally, that it has no repercussions on your general health.

As already said, all sexual activity carries some element of risk – this is not something which has changed recently. For women there has always been the risk of pregnancy, the risks involved in contraception; for both men and women the risk of infection has always been around. However, whether people acknowledge these risks is another matter.

If two people enter into a relationship as openly and as honestly as possible, there is no blame to be apportioned if that other person gets herpes; neglect, blame and guilt flourish only when there is a lack of trust on both sides.

So, to summarise:

- Know your facts about herpes in relation to yourself.
- Examine your own feelings about having herpes.

WHERE TO GO FOR INFORMATION AND SUPPORT

Chapter 6 discusses where to go for diagnosis and treatment. But many people with herpes know how to recognise their attacks and what to do during them; what they want is current information and support.

Most genitourinary clinics have health advisers who are experienced in health education and counselling; you can either see them when you come in for a check-up, or with a separate appointment. They offer not only practical advice, but also more long-term support if you are upset and anxious about herpes.

The clinic nurses are also involved in health education. Many clinics have a walk-in system so that if you don't actually want a check-up, but would like some advice, you can be seen by one of the nurses.

Some family planning and well-women workers are experienced in sexually transmitted infections and counselling, so it's worth airing your anxieties with them. At the very least they will be able to advise you on who to see.

There is also a self-help organisation called the Herpes Association, based in London, but with local groups. They offer practical information about the infection, updates on research work, and support other people with herpes. The Association has a helpline (071-609 9081) as well as a quarterly newsletter (see page 76 for address).

Psychology departments of district hospitals are also involved in counselling. If you want to talk to them you can be referred to a clinical psychologist by your GP, but it's also possible to self refer – health advisers at the STD clinics should be able to tell you how to go about this. The advisers also have information on good counsellors and psychotherapists, as will local community health councils and the British Association for Counselling. It's always worthwhile getting someone else's recommendation, as you will have to pay for most non-statutory counselling services, and there is a plethora of different 'schools' of counselling to choose from (see Useful Addresses).

5

TREATMENT

The treatment of most medical conditions usually involves a number of strategies, including:

- Symptomatic treatment – drugs to treat the symptoms, e.g. pain.
- Specific treatment – drugs to treat the condition itself.
- And self-help – things you can do for yourself.

With genital herpes all three approaches are important.

In this chapter we will review the development of specific anti-herpes drugs, and their use in the treatment of primary and recurrent herpes; symptomatic therapy; the management of some of the complications associated with herpes, including meningitis, sacral radiculomyelopathy, urinary problems, non-genital skin blisters and sores; the management of herpes in pregnancy; the use of other drugs and alternative remedies; and finally the development and possible uses of vaccines. The role of self-help is reviewed in Chapter 6.

SPECIFIC ANTI-HERPES DRUGS

In 1959 researchers who were looking for drugs to treat cancer produced a drug called idoxuridine (Herpid, Iduridin, Virudox). The drug had marked antiviral activity against several viruses including *Herpes simplex.* Idoxuridine works by stopping the virus from reproducing itself, but unfortunately it also stops human cells from dividing which means that it is a very toxic drug causing serious side effects.

It has to be given by injection, it does not work by mouth, and topical idoxuridine (that is, cream or ointment) does not appear to be very successful in treating genital herpes.

Acyclovir

Since 1959 several other anti-herpes drugs have been produced, but most have had limited use because of their serious side effects. However, the introduction of acyclovir (Zovirax), a specific, safe and highly efficacious drug, has revolutionised treatment of genital herpes.

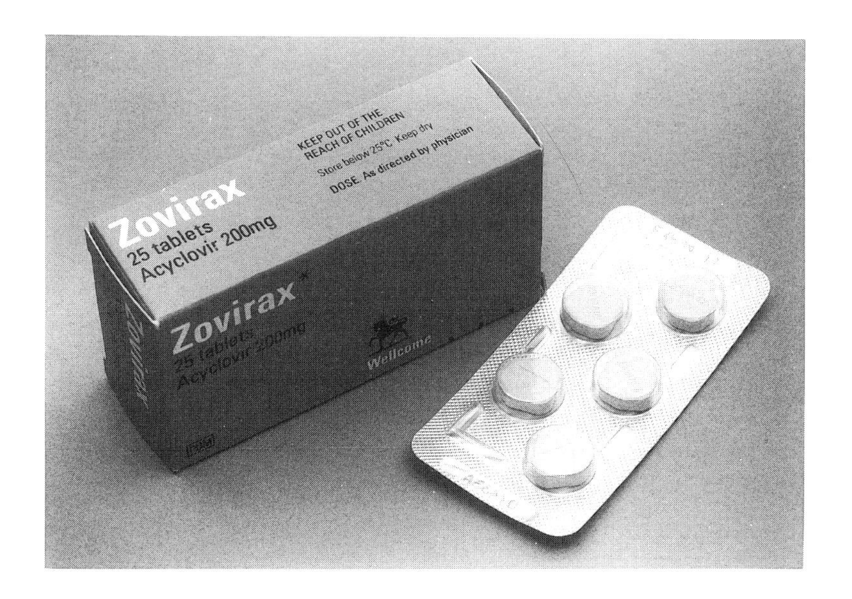

Acyclovir depends for its action on suppression of viral reproduction. This is achieved by a unique mechanism whereby the drug is incorporated into the DNA (the genetic material at the heart of the virus) within infected cells and not the DNA in uninfected human cells. The incorporated drug blocks the step-by-step construction of the strands of viral DNA and thus, stops further viral reproduction. As a result of the selective incorporation into viral DNA, but not human DNA, the drug is very safe.

When to use acyclovir

Acyclovir is a very useful drug for patients with first-attack genital herpes. It allows patients to heal more quickly, it shortens the duration of symptoms including pain in the genital area and on urination, fever, headaches and the flu-like symptoms common with the first attack, and finally it decreases the time during which infectious virus is produced. The drug is particularly useful if started soon (two or three days) after the first blisters have developed; once the sores have started

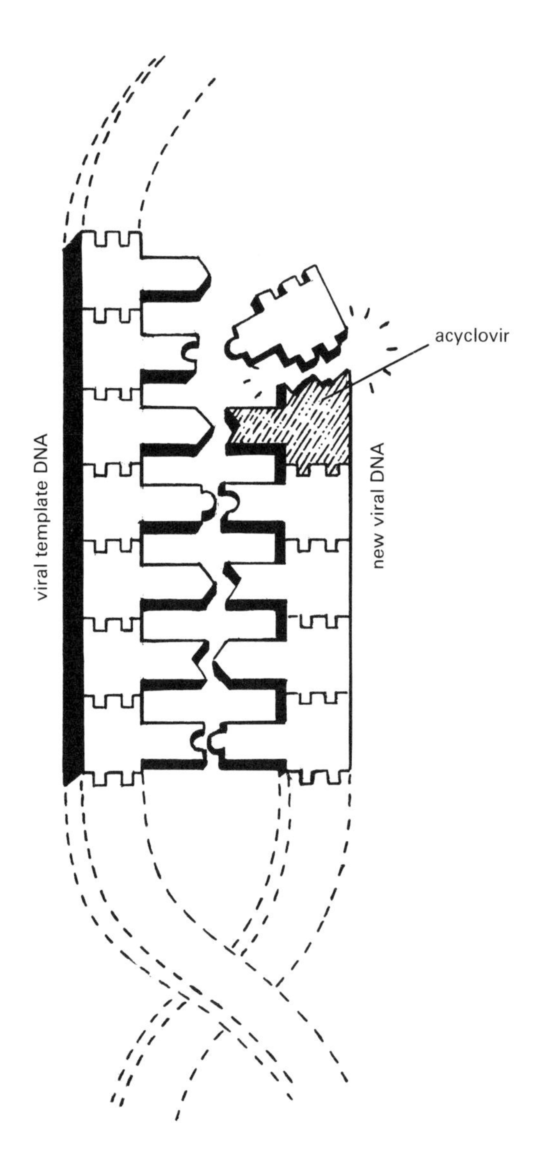

A new strand of viral DNA is being made on the right to complement the template on the left. Once acyclovir has blocked the new sequence on the right, further building blocks cannot enter, thus terminating the DNA chain.

healing, the drug is of limited use. Clinical trials have shown that oral (by mouth) therapy is better than cream or ointment, the recommended dose being one tablet five times daily for five days.

The drug does not cure herpes, it merely shortens the first attack and reduces its severity. Subsequent recurrences (both in terms of frequency and severity) are not affected because latency is believed to be established very early on, and certainly before treatment is started (see Chapter 1). Most people are treated with oral therapy as outpatients, but occasionally if the pain is very severe or there is urinary retention or meningitis, hospital admission may be recommended and acyclovir given by injection into a vein in the arm.

Treatment of each recurrence with acyclovir (either cream or tablets) is useful in some patients, particularly those who have prodromal (warning) symptoms, e.g. pain or tingling, preceding every attack. In these circumstances some patients find that the drug shortens the duration and severity of that particular episode. Unfortunately, though, the majority of people find that the drug is of limited use in this situation and that at best the duration and severity of the recurrences is only very slightly reduced. And some people find that, after a short period of time using the drug during the prodromal phase, recurrences begin to develop without any warning symptoms.

In recent years it has been discovered that there is an alternative method of using acyclovir which is highly successful in patients with frequent recurrences. This involves taking acyclovir tablets every day to prevent the infection from recurring. This treatment is called suppressive or prophylactic treatment, and is particularly useful for people with very frequent recurrences (six or more a year), although it may also be used for those with less frequent, but more prolonged or severe episodes. As mentioned above, acyclovir is a very safe drug and there appear to be no serious long-term adverse effects, even after taking treatment for several years. True, a few patients may experience nausea or minor skin rashes; however, these are usually transient and resolve within a few days.

Most people who are considered suitable for suppressive acyclovir will commence treatment on four tablets daily and over the coming months the dose will be reduced to three or even two tablets a day. The fewer the number of tablets taken each day, the greater the likelihood of having a recurrence, so we generally maintain people on the lowest daily dose which keeps them recurrence free. Several clinical trials have shown that when treatment is stopped, after a short period of time (three to four months) the recurrences return with the same frequency and severity as they were before treatment commenced. However, after longer periods of time (one to two years), the frequency of recurrences after stopping therapy is sometimes markedly reduced. Therefore it is usually recommended that treatment is stopped after a year to determine whether further long-term suppression is necessary.

The majority of patients on long-term suppressive acyclovir will have either no recurrences or very few minor short-lived episodes. There are several additional benefits, including a dramatic reduction in the prodromal symptoms, a marked improvement in psychological well being (in many situations leading to a dramatic improvement in the sexual difficulties associated with herpes), and there may even be a reduction in some of the scars or marks left on the skin from previous recurrences.

There are some disadvantages to treatment. Firstly, it requires a commitment to take the tablets regularly; secondly, it should be stressed that this is a treatment, not a cure; and finally, as with many drugs, acyclovir should not be taken during pregnancy or if one is contemplating falling pregnant.

Suppressive acyclovir is expensive (approximately £1 per tablet at 1990 prices); consequently general practitioners and genitourinary medicine clinics may, because of financial constraints, find it difficult to recommend such treatment for all patients, and this situation is likely to become more acute with the advent of clinical budgeting. If your GP or clinic are having difficulties it may be worth finding another GP or switching to another genitourinary medicine clinic more willing to consider treatment.

Future antiviral drugs

Over the coming years it is extremely likely that a number of new antiviral drugs will be produced. Most will probably be similar to acyclovir, but some may have the advantage that you can take them less frequently, particularly when used for suppression of frequent recurrences.

SYMPTOMATIC TREATMENT

A great deal can be done to relieve the symptoms associated with genital herpes.

Pain relief

The pain associated with first-attack genital herpes may be severe and last several weeks, so the routine use of analgesics (medicines to relieve the pain) is often helpful; two tablets of aspirin or paracetamol every four to six hours, as necessary, are the two drugs most often used. Very occasionally stronger drugs such as pethidine are required; these will always be given under direct medical supervision.

A number of self-help techniques can also be used to relieve the pain, including frequent salt-water bathing and avoidance of tight or restrictive clothing (see Chapter 6 for full discussion).

Control of urinary problems

In patients with severe urinary problems (mostly women), relief from the pain is sometimes enough to allow urination to occur normally. As described in Chapter 6, saline bathing or urination in the bath or simple separation of the labia to stop the urine coming into contact with the sores may also help.

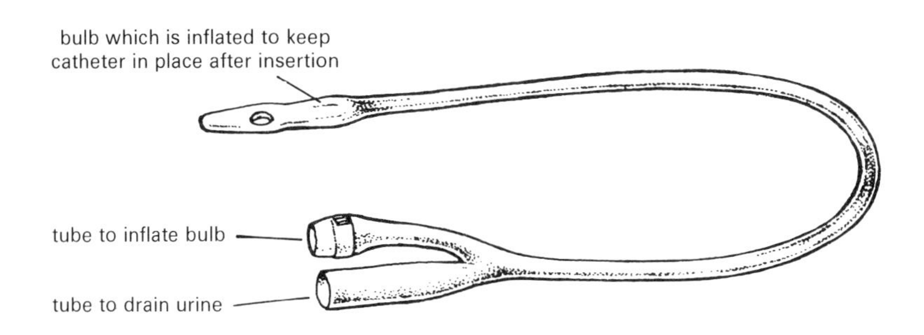

Urethral catheter.

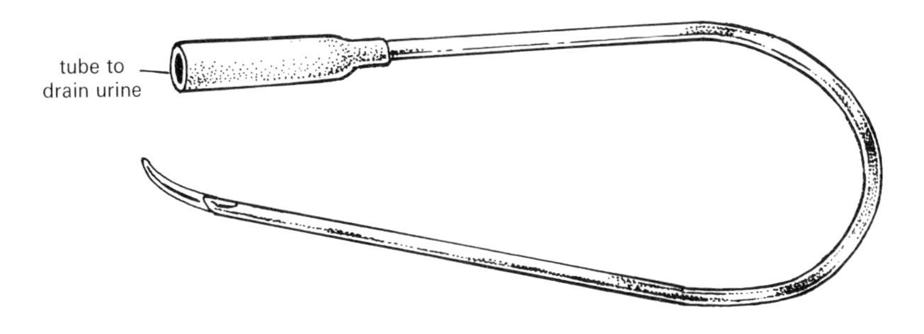

Suprapubic catheter

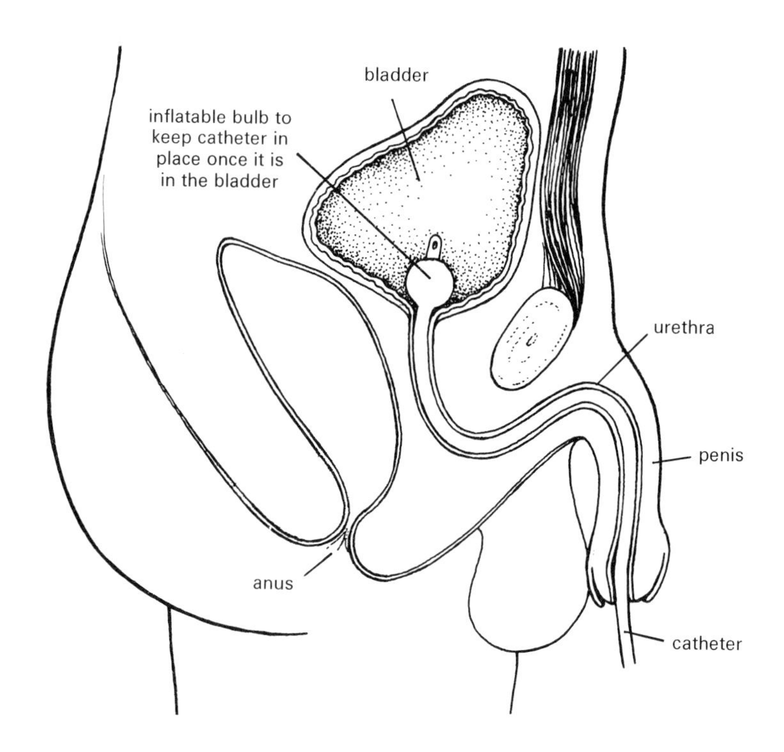

How a urethral catheter is inserted.

Occasionally, the person may be totally unable to pass urine despite all the manoeuvres mentioned above. This occurs particularly if there is an associated sacral radiculomyelopathy (for full discussion see Chapter 3). In these circumstances a catheter (a thin rubber tube) may have to be passed into the bladder to drain the urine, but this procedure is only used if all else fails. Sometimes the catheter will be passed through the urethra (as above), but if there is too much pain or ulceration it may even have to be passed through the lower part of the abdomen into the bladder; this is called a suprapubic catheter (see opposite and on page 70). In most circumstances the catheter may be removed without problems after two to three days.

Treatment of meningitis

Patients who develop meningitis in association with genital herpes will usually be treated with acyclovir. In addition, analgesics and bed rest will almost always be recommended. Symptoms usually settle within a few days.

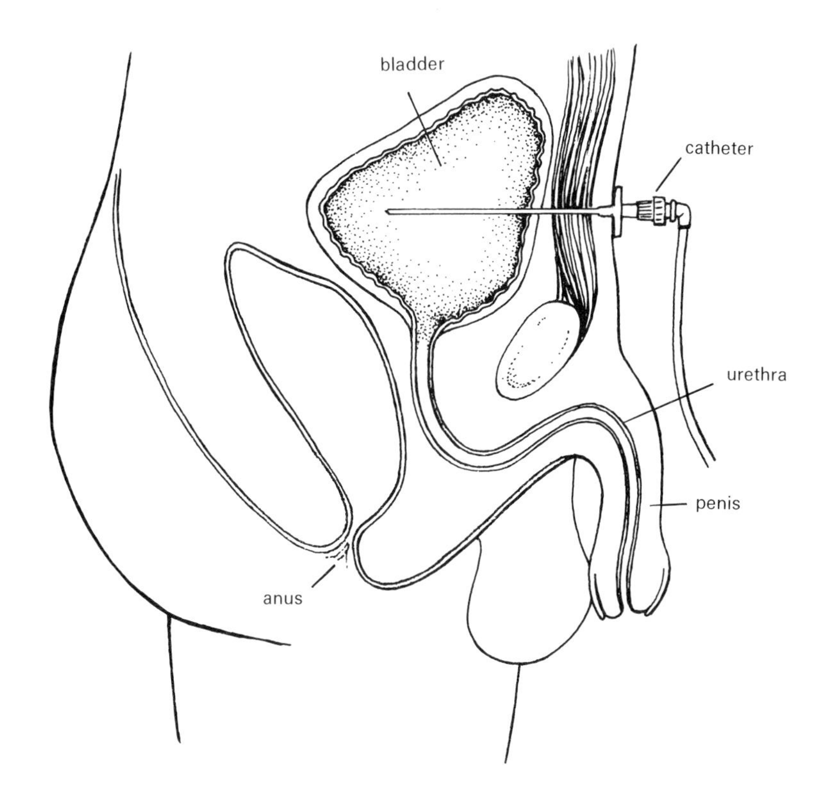

How a suprapubic catheter is inserted.

Treatment of non-genital blisters or sores

Non-genital herpes, for example on the buttock, thigh or hand, may be very painful. Infrequent outbreaks require only symptomatic treatment (analgesics and saline bathing), but people with frequent episodes may benefit from long-term suppressive oral acyclovir (see above). Treating each recurrence with acyclovir, cream or tablets, is of limited value.

HERPES IN PREGNANCY

Herpes infection in newborn babies – neonatal herpes – may result in serious or indeed life-threatening disease, with up to 60 per cent of babies dying and many of the survivors having severe brain damage or damage to other internal organs.

As mentioned in Chapter 3, the infection is usually acquired by the newborn baby either as a result of infection in the mother at the time of delivery or, less commonly, as a consequence of spread across the placenta early in pregnancy. The risk of spread at the time of delivery is greatest in women with primary genital herpes.

Neonatal herpes can be treated with acyclovir. The drug certainly decreases the number of babies who die as a result of the infection, but many of those that survive have serious brain damage. This is probably because the treatment is sometimes started too late (the condition may be very difficult to diagnose in the newborn) and also because the treatment appears to be less effective in the newborn, perhaps because the baby's immune system is not fully developed. Prevention of the infection in the newborn remains a priority.

Women with primary genital herpes

If a woman has primary genital herpes at or around the onset of labour, many obstetricians would recommend a Caesarean section in order that the baby can bypass the infected birth canal. Caesarean section is usually successful in preventing neonatal infection, but unfortunately a small number of babies are infected despite this procedure. This is usually because the infection spreads to the baby as a consequence of prolonged rupture of the membranes or, very rarely, as a result of spread from the mother's blood through the placenta to the baby. Caesarean section is not without risk as the procedure involves a major abdominal operation and an anaesthetic and, whilst this is a routine procedure, problems do occasionally occur.

Recently there has been interest in the use of acyclovir for pregnant women with primary genital herpes around the time of birth. Most doctors (and indeed pregnant women) are reluctant to use any drugs in pregnancy for fear of causing damage to the baby; however, acyclovir has been used in a small number of women with severe primary genital herpes at term with no apparent ill effects in either the mother or the baby. Further information is required before this form of treatment can be widely used.

Fortunately, primary genital herpes is rare in pregnancy, and consequently neonatal infection acquired in this way is also very unusual.

Women with recurrent genital herpes

If a woman with a history of recurrent genital herpes has an active herpetic lesion at the time of delivery, there is a remote chance that the baby will be infected on its passage through the birth canal (see Chapter 3).

Because this risk is small there is considerable controversy surrounding the management of this problem. Most obstetricians recommend that if a woman with a history of recurrent genital herpes has an open herpetic sore near the vaginal entrance at the time of onset of labour a Caesarean section should be performed. In order to detect sores, women are often asked to come back to the clinic every week from 36 weeks of pregnancy until the onset of labour so that the genitals may be carefully inspected. In our opinion this is a useful procedure as it allows the doctors and midwives to detect early sores and the woman herself to report any symptoms possibly associated with early herpes. Some doctors also recommend that swabs for viral cultures should be taken from the cervix and vulva every week from 36 weeks of pregnancy until delivery, in order to detect asymptomatic viral shedding (see Chapter 2). However the value of this latter procedure has been questioned on the grounds that the results of the tests are not usually available for at least a week and consequently the information obtained is of little value.

As mentioned above, if a woman with recurrent herpes has an obvious herpetic sore near the vaginal entrance at the time of the onset of labour a Caesarean section is recommended. However, if lesions are well away from the vaginal entrance a normal vaginal delivery may be permitted. Recently, there has been considerable interest in the possible use of acyclovir to prevent reaction of herpes in pregnancy, thereby avoiding the necessity for Caesarean section and infection in the baby. Studies are underway to see if acyclovir can be given in late pregnancy to stop genital herpes from occurring and consequently the baby from being infected. Another suggested approach is to treat all babies who may have been exposed to the virus during delivery with acyclovir. It should be stressed that these procedures are experimental and considerably more information concerning the safety of acyclovir in pregnancy and its usefulness are required before these forms of treatment can be recommended.

It should be emphasised again that neonatal herpes is very rare and that the risk to the newborn baby from a mother with recurrent genital herpes is very slight, whatever procedure is adopted for screening or treatment. The recent introduction of blood tests to detect type-specific herpes antibodies may enable the doctor to predict which women are at risk of infecting their babies; studies using these tests are awaited with interest. (For a full discussion see Chapter 2.)

OTHER TREATMENTS

The accompanying box lists some of the treatments which have been used or suggested for use in the treatment of genital herpes. Some, including the antivirals, are conventional drugs, others are not. Many of the conventional treatments have been evaluated in carefully controlled clinical trials, whereas the majority of alternative remedies have not.

Treatments which have been used or suggested for use with genital herpes

Antivirals	Idoxuridine (Herpid, Iduridin, Virudox) Acyclovir (Zovirax)
Antiseptics and spermicides	Ether Betadine Methyl alcohol Gentian violet Copper sulphate Potassium permanganate Nonoxynol-9
Immune modulators	Inosine pranobex (Imunovir) Interferons Vaccines
Antibiotics	Co-trimoxazole (Septrin, Bactrim, Comox, Laratrim)
Miscellaneous	Vitamins (E, C, B_{12}) Lithium Zinc Gingseng *Aloe vera* extracts Red algae L-lysine

Antiseptic and spermicides

Several antiseptics have been shown to be able to damage or even kill viruses when tested in the laboratory, and consequently have been suggested as useful preparations for the treatment of genital herpes. The majority of these preparations have not been evaluated in clinical trials, though, and it seems unlikely that they are able to penetrate the skin or mucous membranes and destroy the virus within cells. None the less, some people find them useful.

Spermicides, such as nonoxynol-9 have also been shown to have some antiviral activity when tested in the laboratory. While it is possible that the use of these chemicals, either in the form of spermicide jellies or as lubricants on condoms, may help to decrease the risk of transmission of herpes, they are of no use for the treatment of the condition.

Immune modulators

These are drugs that increase or boost the immune response to herpes, and include naturally occurring products such as the interferons (Chapter 1) and other drugs which are said to boost the various cells within the immune system including the natural killer cells, macrophages and lymphocytes (see Chapter 1). Clinical trials have not shown any convincing evidence that any of these drugs have any use for the treatment of genital herpes, and most are not available for its treatment.

One drug, inosine pranobex (Imunovir) is available in the United Kingdom and Europe. Although early studies suggested that this drug was useful for the treatment of genital herpes, more recent trials comparing acyclovir with inosine pranobex have shown that the former is superior to the latter in all aspects of treatment. Although inosine pranobex is still occasionally recommended, our own feeling is that it has no place in the treatment of genital herpes.

In the past doctors treating herpes have used a variety of vaccines against other infections, including yellow fever, tuberculosis and influenza, in an attempt to give a general boost to the body's immune system and thereby possibly decrease the frequency of herpes recurrences. However there is no evidence that this strategy works, and it has largely been abandoned.

There have also been attempts to produce a vaccine against genital herpes (this is discussed in detail below). Some of these vaccines have been used in people with recurrent genital herpes in an attempt to reduce the frequency and severity of recurrences, but here again there is no convincing evidence that this helps in any way and we would not recommend their use.

Antibiotics

Antibiotics (drugs that kill bacteria or stop them reproducing) are sometimes recommended for the treatment of herpes, the reason for doing this being that bacteria that normally live on the skin or mucous membranes may occasionally cause problems where the skin is broken or ulcerated. But this problem only occurs very rarely, and even if it does the immune system is usually capable of coping with it. As a consequence, antibiotics are rarely if ever useful for the treatment of genital herpes.

Miscellaneous therapies

There are numerous and diverse miscellaneous remedies that have been recommended for the treatment of herpes. Some are based on laboratory evidence of antiviral efficacy and some on case reports in the medical literature. In many, including the vitamins, ginseng and *Aloe vera* extracts, there is no apparent scientific evidence that these preparations have any effect on the infection.

There has been considerable interest in the use of L-lysine, which is a chemical called an amino acid. Amino acids occur naturally in foodstuffs and are the building blocks for proteins, the chemicals that, among other things, control all the metabolic events in the body. Experiments in the laboratory suggested that L-lysine could inhibit the reproduction of *Herpes simplex* virus, but clinical trials have not substantiated this claim. Despite this, many people believe that the balance of L-lysine and arginine (another amino acid) is important in the prevention or reduction of recurrences. Foods high in L-lysine, e.g. fresh fish, goats' milk, cheese, eggs, brewers' yeast and many beans, are believed to reduce attacks, whilst those high in arginine, e.g. nuts, chickpeas and rice, make them worse. In addition, some people report that additional L-lysine, in the form of capsules, may also help. We do not believe that L-lysine has any effect on genital herpes; however, if you find it useful we see no reason why you should not continue, as there are unlikely to be any adverse effects.

VACCINES FOR HERPES

A vaccine is a chemical (usually a protein) derived from a virus or bacteria which is given to a person who has not been exposed to that particular infection; it causes the immune system to respond by developing a defence against that particular virus or bacteria, and thus protects the person against subsequently developing that infection. There are numerous vaccines against many diverse infections (for example smallpox, tuberculosis, polio and tetanus, to mention but a few).

Over recent years there has been considerable interest in the possible development of vaccines against herpes. Several potential vaccines have been produced, mostly derived from the glycoproteins on the envelope of the virus (see Chapter 1), and some have been shown to be capable of protecting laboratory animals against infection. Some of these vaccines have been tested in humans and various claims concerning their efficacy have been made. Unfortunately, there is no convincing scientific evidence that any of those thus far produced have any effect. Carefully conducted clinical trials to establish the safety and usefulness of these vaccines are now urgently needed.

It is possible that a vaccine capable of protecting people from *Herpes simplex* virus may be available in the not too distant future. However, even if such a vaccine is produced, it should be remembered that the majority of people exposed to herpes never develop any clinical problems, and in most of those who do the problems are minimal. This is unlike the situation with many other infections, e.g. smallpox or polio, where there are serious or life threatening consequences. As a result any herpes vaccine will only have limited use.

6

WHERE TO GO AND WHAT TO DO

This chapter will discuss where to go and what to do if you think you have genital herpes.

WHERE TO GO

If you have any of the symptoms discussed in Chapter 2 it's important that you have a check-up to confirm the diagnosis, that you're given the appropriate information and, if necessary, treatment. There are several places you can visit.

- Genito-urinary clinics.
- Your GP.
- Family planning/well-women clinics.
- Accident and emergency department at your local district general hospital.

You will find the number of your nearest family planning or well-women clinic in the phone book, or alternatively phone the Family Planning Association (see Useful addresses). However it should be remembered that neither these clinics, nor a GP's surgery usually have the facilities to take specimens for subsequent tests.

If you can't be seen by your GP or at any of the clinics, and if your symptoms worsen, especially at night or at the weekend, you can always visit your nearest accident and emergency department. This is really only relevant if it is your first attack, or if you are immunocompromised, i.e. if your immune system is not functioning properly because you are HIV antibody positive, have AIDS or are being treated with chemotherapy or radiotherapy for any illness, and are suffering severe recurrences.

It is important that wherever you go, if you have symptoms at the time, you are examined by the doctor.

A GU clinic

However the most appropriate place to visit if you have, or think you have, a sexually transmitted infection is a genito-urinary clinic. In the past these have variously been called VD, STD and special clinics. You should be able to find them listed in the telephone book under 'Venereal' – they are usually in, or attached to, hospitals. Libraries, GP surgeries, family planning clinics, listings magazines all usually have the name and telephone number of the clinics in your area. It is important to telephone first if you can, because some clinics run appointment systems. Opening times can also be varied.

These clinics are governed by different legislation from other outpatient departments, so that the public has direct access; that is, you don't need a referral letter from your GP. It should be emphasised that all information you give in a GU clinic is completely confidential, that no information will be sent to your GP unless you were referred by them in the first place or you request the clinic to do so. It's also worth remembering that all investigations and medication prescribed in a GU clinic are free. The work there includes screening, diagnosing and treating sexually transmitted infections and other genital complaints.

When you visit a GU clinic you will usually be interviewed initially by a doctor to ascertain what the problem is. They will also ask you questions about your general health, contraceptive practices, sexuality, and sexual behaviour, including safer sex and HIV. A clinical examination then follows.

Routine screening in genito-urinary clinics

Females	*Males*
Thrush	Non-specific urethritis (NSU) (including chlamydia)
Anaerobic vaginosis	Gonorrhoea
Trichomonas (TV)	Warts
Gonorrhoea	Syphilis
Chlamydia	
Warts	
Syphilis	

Females – routine clinical examination

If you are seen by a male doctor you will usually be chaperoned by a nurse. The clinical examination, and taking of specimens, takes about 10 minutes. All new patients receive this routine screening; so whether it is your first attack or a recurrence, it is recommended that you have this done.

There are four parts to a routine examination:

- Examination of external genitals. In order to be examined it is necessary to lie in the same position as you would for any gynaecological procedure, including smears, cap and coil fitting. The doctor will then carefully check the area, from your pubis at the front of your genitals to your anus at the back, for any redness, itching, blisters, ulceration, or what may look like cuts or abrasion – in fact anything not normally there.

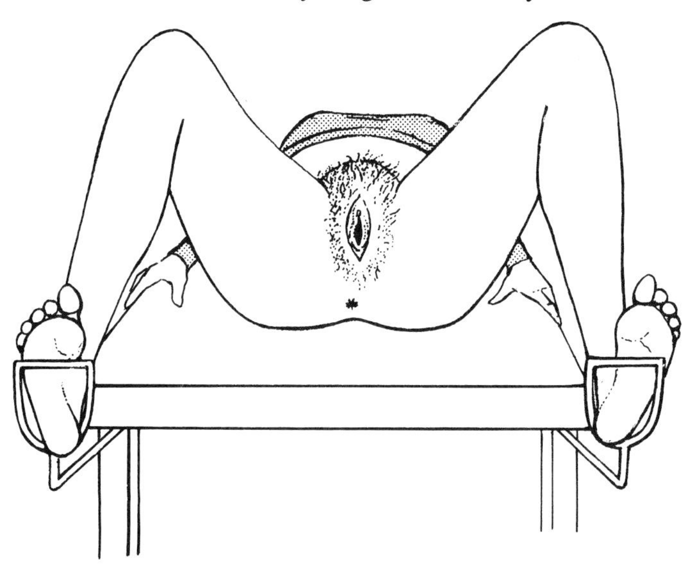

How an external examination is made.

- Examination of your internal genitalis – the 'internal'. A speculum will be inserted and opened in order to allow the doctor to examine your vaginal walls and cervix, which are the commonest sites for other sexually transmitted infections. As well as again checking for any abnormalities, the doctor will take swabs of vaginal, cervical and urethral secretions. These will then be examined for evidence of other infections. If you have extensive ulceration and it is too swollen and painful to insert a speculum, the doctor will defer the internal examination until you're better.

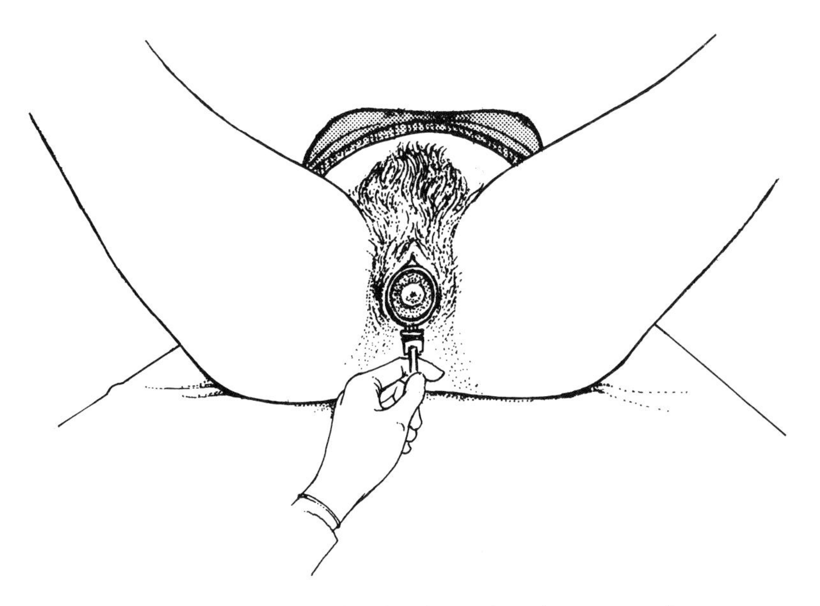

How an internal vaginal examination is made using a speculum.

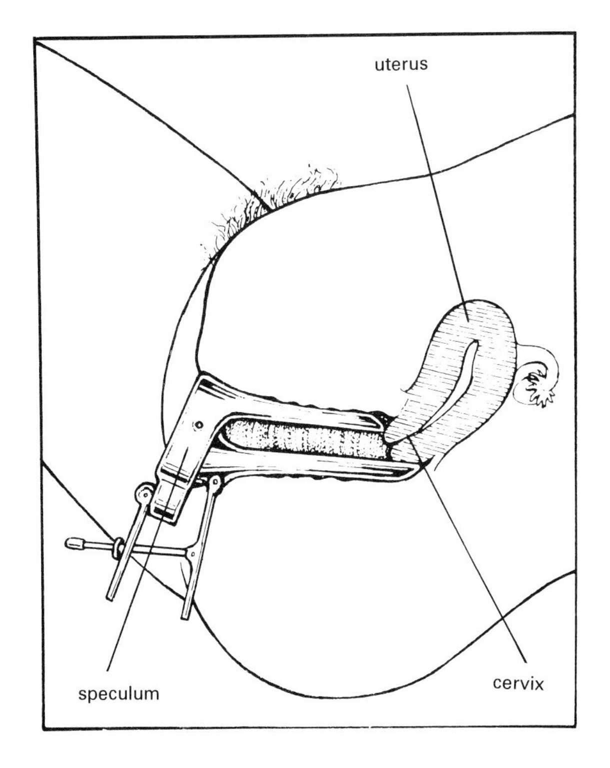

Speculum in place during a vaginal examination.

- A small sample of blood is taken, to check for syphillis. Blood to test for HIV antibodies is only taken at the patient's request, and after counselling. However, HIV and safer sex may be discussed during your interview with the doctor.
- Finally you will be asked to produce a small sample of urine.

If you've had oral or anal sex it's important to tell the doctor, as extra swabs may need to be taken from these sites.

Males – routine clinical examination

This depends on the type of sexual activity you've been having, and where you've noticed symptoms.

- If you've had oral sex your mouth and throat will be examined and swabs taken from the back of the throat as it is not uncommon for infection from the vagina, penis or anus to be transmitted to this area during oral sex.
- If you've had unprotected sex (that is, without using a condom), whether vaginal, anal or oral, and have a urethral discharge from the tip of the penis, or a burning or tingling sensation on passing urine, a swab will be taken by passing a tiny loop into the urethra. This may feel uncomfortable, but not painful. You will then be asked to pass urine.

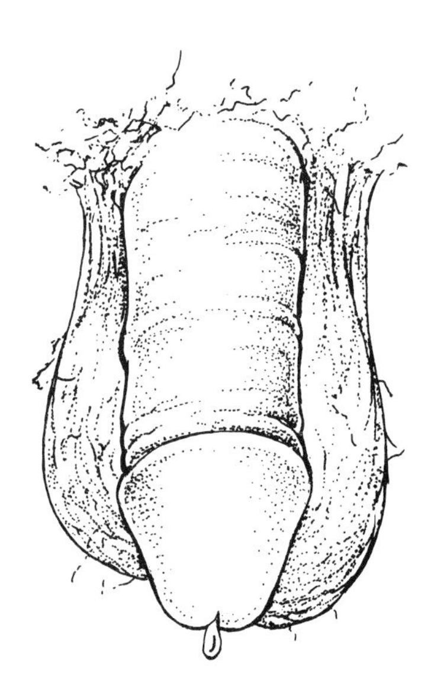

Discharge from tip of the penis.

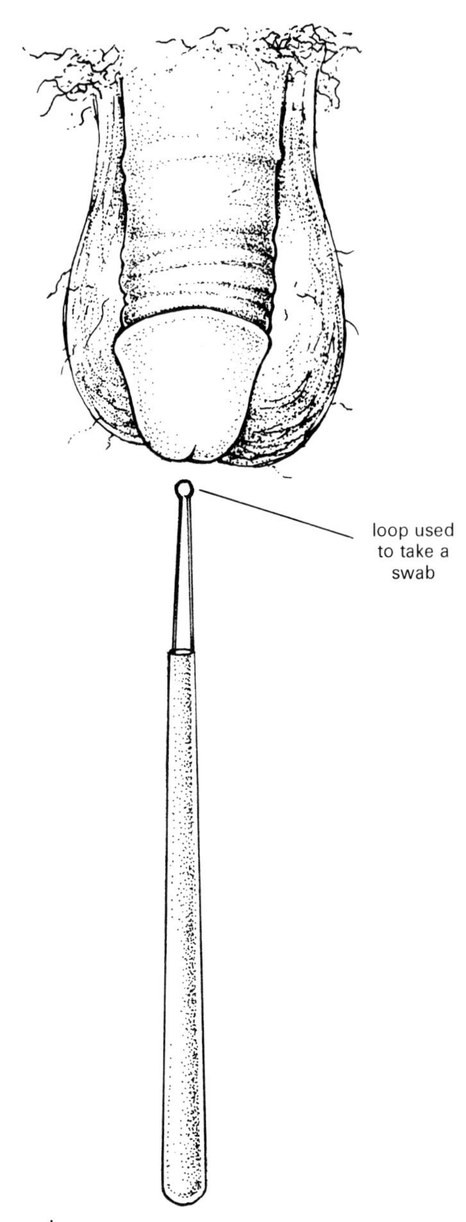

Taking a urethral swab.

- If you have had unprotected anal intercourse, i.e. if your partner(s) have not used condoms, swabs may well be taken from the anorectal canal – the back passage. This involves passing into the anus a small instrument called a proctoscope, which enables the doctor to visualise and examine the area.

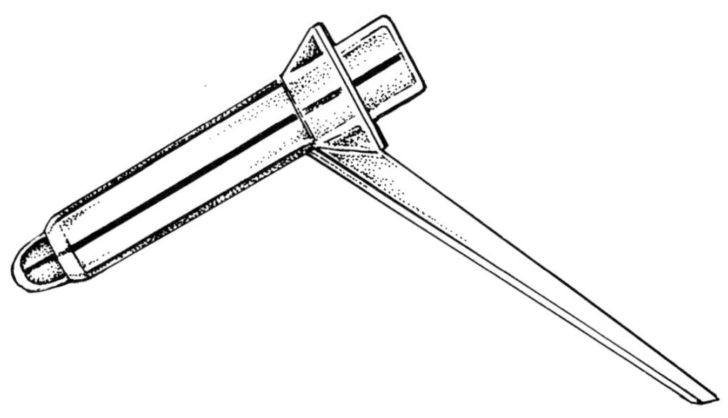

Proctoscope used for anal examination.

- A blood sample will be taken to test for syphilis. As with the female examination, blood to test for HIV antibodies is only taken at the patient's request and after counselling. However, HIV and safer sex may be discussed by the doctor during the initial interview.

Testing for herpes

As you can see from the table on page 61, herpes is not part of a routine screening; herpes cannot be diagnosed from vaginal/urethral secretions, nor is there a blood test to detect it (see Chapter 2). Instead it is diagnosed from:

- The history you give the doctor (see previous chapters for the signs and symptoms).
- A careful examination of the genitals.
- A positive viral culture.

To take a specimen for a viral culture a cotton bud is pressed firmly into the lesion; this may be painful, but takes only seconds. A positive culture then means that, under laboratory conditions, herpes virus is found in the sample taken. However, unlike in other infections, a negative culture does not always mean that you don't have herpes: it can mean that not enough virus was being shed from the site where the swab was taken. If you have already started antiviral medication before your examination, this is also likely to cause a negative result.

Many GU clinics have workers called health advisers who are experienced in health education and counselling. You should be offered the opportunity to discuss herpes with them, whether you've come to the clinic with a first outbreak or a recurrence.

Why test for other diseases?

You will be given the results of some tests at the initial visit, but another appointment will be made at which you can receive the other results. It is most important that you are aware of these, in case treatment is necessary.

But why, if you've come to the clinic for a specific reason, is it recommended that you have a full screening for other sexually transmitted infections? There are two reasons.

- By putting yourself at risk of one sexually transmitted infection you are also at risk of exposure to other infections contracted through sexual activity.
- The symptoms of some infections are often similar and can mask other infections. Some vaginal thrush can be severe and painful, just as some outbreaks of herpes can be very small and look like tiny skin abrasions. Some infections like chlamydia often have no symptoms at all. And, whereas herpes has no long-term ill effects, untreated chlamydia or gonorrhoea in women can create serious problems with fertility.

It is therefore common sense to include/exclude the possibility of other infections.

WHAT TO DO

The next part of the chapter will discuss what to do when you have a first episode, and then what to do if and when you have a recurrence.

What to do during a first episode

- You may feel systemically, i.e. generally, unwell – headache, backache, flu-like symptoms, drained of all energy. The best thing to do is, after you've seen the doctor, go home and rest until you feel better. Leave the affected area exposed. If you work, you may need to take a couple of days off.
- Depending on the severity of the outbreak, your doctor may well treat you with the antiviral drug acyclovir (see Chapter 5). This will not cure herpes, nor will it remove the possibility of a recurrence: however it will reduce the length and severity of the attack. As with any drugs, it's important to tell the doctor if you think you may be pregnant.
- Whilst you're resting, an ice pack, or a packet of frozen

peas (they mould easily), applied to the genitals can have a soothing anaesthetic effect.

- Mild analgesics (painkillers) like paracetamol or aspirin may relieve the discomfort, especially if you're experiencing pain or aching down the legs.
- Salt water helps to dry up the ulcers and is quite soothing – put half a cup of ordinary salt in a bath. If you don't have a bath, pouring warm salty water over the affected area is just as effective.
- Try and wear loose, preferably cotton, clothing whilst you're up and about.
- For many women it can be painful passing urine. What happens is that the acidic urine comes into contact with the delicate broken skin, so it's not surprising that it's painful. If you can, sit in a bath to urinate, which will not only reduce the discomfort but will also help you to relax. Again, if you don't have a bath, you could either squat in a washing up bowl of warm water or, whilst you're on the toilet, pour warm water over your vulva whilst you're urinating.
- Sometimes, especially with a first attack, men may experience pain on passing urine. The best thing to do is drink plenty of bland fluids. However, if you notice a discharge, or a burning sensation, it's important to rule out any other sexually transmitted infections.
- If you have lesions in or around the anus, it may be painful to open your bowels. Plenty of fluids, fruit and vegetables should help in order to avoid constipation – constipation will just make defaecating more painful. You may notice some bleeding when you open your bowels; don't be alarmed, this is because the skin is friable and easily broken.
- From when you experience the first symptoms until the lesions have completely healed, i.e. when any scabs have gone, you should have no close sexual contact with another person. During this time you are infectious, but only if the affected area comes into close skin-to-skin contact with another person. This does not mean no social contact, kissing (if no cold sores), cuddling, etc. (See section on safer sex at the end of this chapter.)
- Basically, leave well alone. Don't put any lotions or potions on the sores – the sooner they dry up, the sooner they will heal. A first episode may take two weeks or longer to heal but it's important to remember that, despite the pain and discomfort, in the majority of people it is self-limiting and leaves no scars. As you can see, medication plays a rela-

tively small part in treating a first attack – it's mainly symptomatic relief.

Herpes and cystitis in women

In women the pain and discomfort on urination is quite often confused with cystitis. However cystitis is generally caused by an infection in the urine or urethra; not only can it be painful to pass water, but there is usually frequency and urgency as well – you need to go to the toilet, sometimes every few minutes, and when you do go you only pass very small amounts of urine.

It is important to differentiate between herpes and cystitis because if you do have a urinary tract infection (cystitis) you may need to take a course of antibiotics, whereas if it is herpes causing the pain you won't want to be treated with antibiotics unnecessarily. Furthermore, if it's cystitis it's also important to drink plenty of bland non-acidic fluids like barley water, to reduce the burning and irritation. A urine sample will normally be tested for a urinary tract infection.

As already mentioned, if you feel you want to pass urine but can't, and it's becoming increasingly uncomfortable, it's important to go to a GU clinic, to your GP or to a casualty department. Very occasionally, either because the urethra becomes swollen or because there is some temporary local nerve interference, you may need to have a catheter (a small rubber tube) passed up your urethra and into your bladder, which will drain the urine and relieve the discomfort. Occasionally, if the urethra has become very swollen and painful, the catheter will be passed directly through the skin, above the pubic line, and then into the bladder (see diagram on next page). It should be stressed that it is uncommon to experience retention of urine, but it's important to be aware of the symptoms (see also Chapter 3 and Chapter 5).

If you have a recurrence

Chapter 2 discusses how to recognise when you are having a recurrence. This section will discuss what to do if you have one, and ways of reducing the frequency of recurrences.

Little is understood as to why some people never have another attack, whilst others have frequent recurrences; no two people have the same pattern. However for many people, if they do have more outbreaks, they are less severe and of a shorter duration than their first episode.

Just as with a first attack, treatment is mainly symptomatic; unless these recurrences become very frequent or severe, there's no need to go to the doctor.

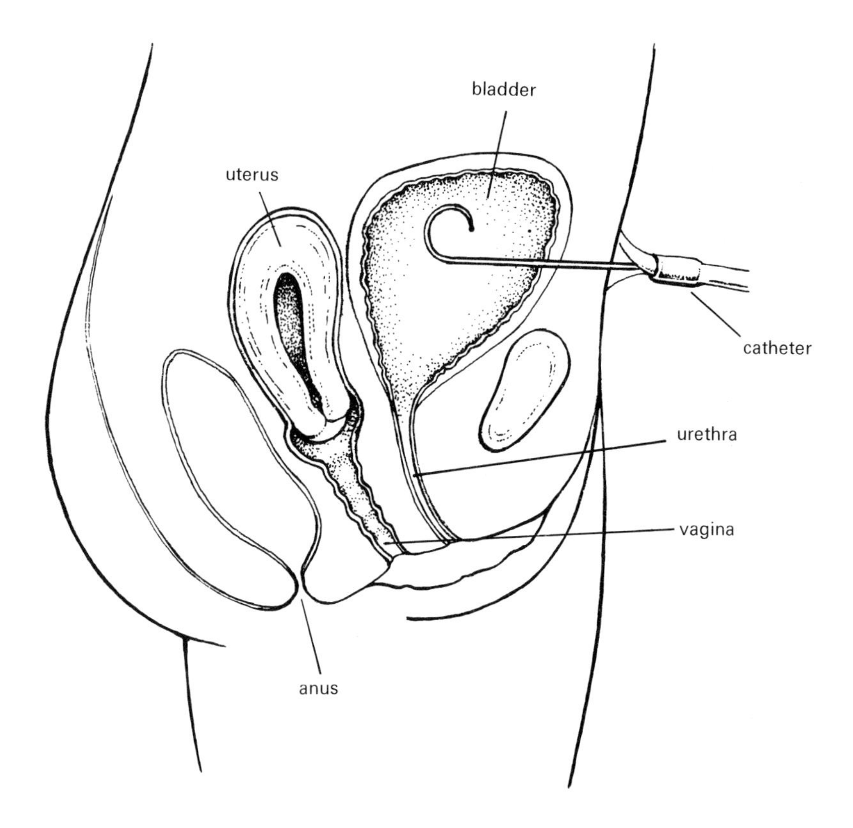

Suprapubic catheter (see also pages 51–2).

- Rest if you can, leaving the area exposed.
- Whilst you're at work, etc., try to wear loose clothing, with cotton underwear. Try not to wear tights which create a warm damp environment which is not conducive to the sores drying up and healing. Stockings or tights without a gusset are preferable.
- Salt-water bathing has a soothing relaxing effect – use half a cup of ordinary salt in the bath. Again if you don't have a bath, either pouring warm salt water over the sores, or dabbing them with salt-water soaked cotton wool helps.
- An ice pack, or a packet of frozen peas, applied to the affected area can be soothing and anaesthetic.
- Mild painkillers like paracetamol or aspirin can relieve the pain and discomfort.
- A hot water bottle can relieve the warning (prodromal) back or groin ache.
- No close sexual contact should occur from the time when

you experience warning symptoms until the lesions (sores) have completely healed.

- There is little benefit in using acyclovir for individual recurrent attacks as it only slightly reduces the duration. (Chapter 5 discusses this in more detail.)

What you do, and what you feel like doing, during a recurrence very much depends on the severity and frequency, but most people who have recurrences learn to recognise signs and symptoms and have their own ways of dealing with them.

For the majority of people who have recurrences, they mostly appear in the same place. However, the nerves from the sacral ganglia cover an area from the base of the spine to the thighs. If you find that attacks start to occur in areas other than usual, say on the buttocks, don't be alarmed and assume that you've reinfected yourself; lesions can occur anywhere in the nerve network. Once you've got the virus, you can't reinfect yourself and, whilst the site of infection may change, as may the frequency or severity, this is the natural history of the virus and not a new infection.

What causes reactivation?

There are some triggers which are thought to reactivate the virus for some people:

- Direct sunlight – whilst you're sunbathing use a good sunblock, and don't expose the area where you usually get attacks. Dry and cracked skin is a good site for a recurrence.
- Sexual intercourse, by the friction involved, can precipitate recurrences, as the skin around the genitals is delicate and friable. It's a good idea to use condoms anyway, and most are lubricated, but extra lubrication like KY Jelly can protect the skin from abrasion. Don't use oil-based lubricants like vaseline with condoms or diaphragms, as they rot the rubber.
- Some women find that they get attacks at the same time as their period, or in mid-cycle. However, taking oral contraception doesn't seem to bring any benefit.

For many people there seems to be no pattern to their recurrences, but they do notice that when they are tired, after an illness, or under pressure at work or home, the frequency of recurrences increases. It would therefore seem sensible to ensure that you maintain a good diet, cut down on smoking, alcohol and drugs, keep to a good balance of relaxation and activity, and try and reduce stress. In this way you might be able to reduce the frequency of attacks.

However this is not always the case and, despite changes in lifestyle, attacks persist. It would also be unrealistic to suggest you can just change your job, or, if you are at home with small children or a sick relative, that you can just walk away from the situation. Having said that, if you're tired, hungover, harassed at work, you'll be less likely to cope well with an attack if you do have one; so that moderation, not denial, would seem a good idea for your physical and mental well being.

SAFER SEX

Safer sex means reducing the risk of contacting and transmitting all sexually transmitted infections. Anyone who is sexually active is at risk of exposure to such infections, from NSU to HIV – the activity involved is the same, unprotected sex, whether it be vaginal, anal or oral.

You can reduce the risk of infection, and this includes exposure to herpes, by the use of condoms; condoms reduce the risk of exchange of body fluids – semen, blood, vaginal fluids – although it is important that the condom is used properly (see diagram opposite). Also check that the condoms you use have a British Standards Kitemark. A diaphragm (the cap) is also a good barrier to infection, although not nearly so effective as a condom. And it is important to remember that any sexual practice, not just penetrative intercourse, that involves exposure to, and exchange of, body fluids should be viewed as carrying a risk.

- Whilst you're having an attack of herpes you should avoid close sexual contact, even when using a condom, from the time when you experience warning symptoms until the lesion has completely healed.
- If you or your sexual partner have cold sores around the mouth, the same applies – you can contract genital herpes from having oral sex with someone with a cold sore.

  As already discussed, the use of condoms can reduce friction and reactivation of attacks in some people. It also reduces the risk of transmission from inapparent attacks.

But you can't transmit or contract herpes:

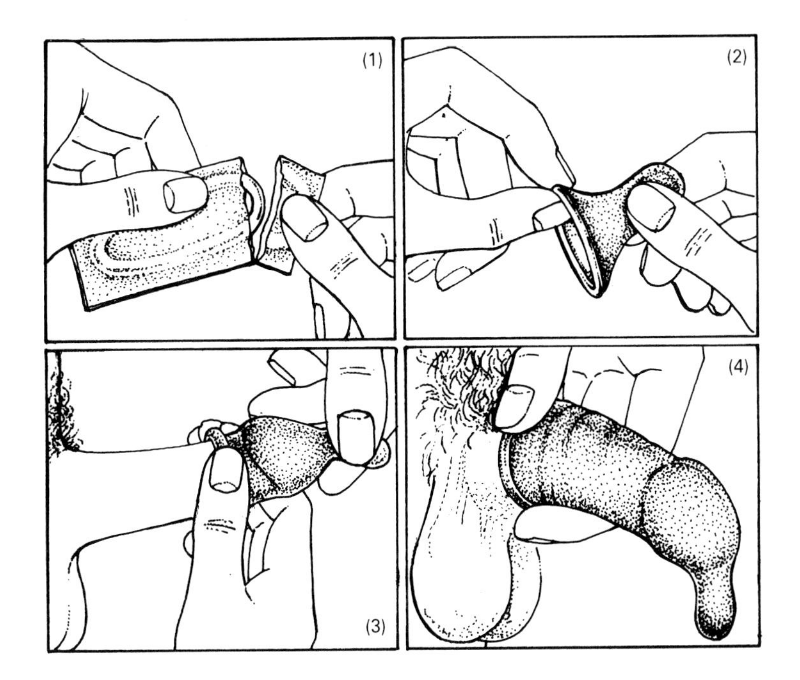

(1) Open packet taking care not to damage the condom.
(2) Squeeze condom tip to expel air.
(3) Gently unroll the condom onto erect penis.
(4) Withdraw penis after ejaculation, holding the condom rim to the base of the penis as you do so.

Correct use of a condom.

- From cups, towels and toilet seats.
- From swimming pools and bath water.
- From blood transfusions – having herpes doesn't mean you can't donate blood.
- If both you and your partner have herpes, you can't reinfect each other.

CONCLUSION

This chapter has been concerned with the practical issues of herpes – what to do and where to go. It can be difficult to gain a perspective on herpes, especially if you have frequent recurrences, or if you feel angry and miserable about it. It is therefore important to know that, not only are there practical ways to minimise its interference in your life; but also that you don't need to feel isolated, that there are others to whom you can turn for information and support.

USEFUL ADDRESSES

Association of Sexual and Marital Therapists
PO Box 62
Sheffield S10 3TS

British Association of Cancer United Patients (BACUP)
121-123 Charterhouse Street
London EC1M 6AA
071-608 1661

British Association for Counselling
37a Sheep Street
Rugby
Warwickshire CV21 3BX
0788 78328/9

Brook Advisory Service
233 Tottenham Court Road
London W1P 9AE
071-323 1522
Your local Brook Advisory Centre will be listed in your phone book.

Citizens' Advice Bureau
Listed under Citizens' Advice Bureau in your phone book.

Community Health Councils
Listed under Community Health Council in your phone book.

Family Planning Information Service
27–35 Mortimer Street
London W1N 7RJ
071-636 7866

Genito-urinary medicine clinics
Also called sexually transmitted disease (STD) clinics, special clinics, venereal disease (VD) clinics.
Look in the phone book under Venereal.

Health Education Authority
78 New Oxford Street
London WC1A 1AH
071-631 0930

Health education units
Look in the phone book under name of your local health authority, under the overall heading of National Health Service.

Health Literature Line
0800 555777

Herpes Association
41 North Road
London N7 9DP
071-609 9061

Jewish Marriage Council
23 Ravenshurst Avenue
London NW4 4EL
081-203 6311

The London Centre for Psychotherapy
19 Fitzjohn's Avenue
London NW3 5JY
071-435 0873

Marie Stopes Centre
10 Queen Square
Leeds LS2 8AJ
0532 440685

Marie Stopes Centre
1 Police St
Manchester M2 7LQ
061-832 4250

Marie Stopes House
The Well Woman Centre
108 Whitfield St
London W1
071-388 0662/2585

National AIDS helpline
0800 567123

National Association of Young People's Counselling and Advisory Services
17-23 Albion Street
Leicester LE1 6GD
0533 558763

National Childbirth Trust
9 Queensborough Terrace
Bayswater
London W2 3TB
071-221 3833

Relate (Formerly, National Marriage Guidance Council)
(head office)
Herbert Gray College
Little Church Street
Rugby
Warwickshire CV21 3AP
0788 73241

Relate Northern Ireland
76 Dublin Road
Belfast BT2 7HP
0232 323454

Scottish AIDS Monitor
0345 090966

Scottish Health Education Group
Woodburn House
Canaan Lane
Edinburgh EH10 4SG
031-447 8044

SPOD
Association to Aid Sexual and Personal Relationships of People with a Disability
286 Camden Road
London N7 0BJ

Terrence Higgins Trust
BM AIDS
London WC1N 3XX
071-242 1010

Women Against Cervical Cancer (WACC)
86 Beaufort Street
London SW3 6BU
071-352 1440

Women's Health Concern
17 Earl's Terrace
London W8 6LP
081-602 6669

Women's Health Information Centre
52 Featherstone Street
London EC1
071-251 6580

Women's National Cancer Control Campaign
1 South Audley Street
London W1Y 5DQ
071-495 4995

Women's Reproductive Rights Information Centre
52-54 Featherstone Street
London EC1Y 8RT
071-251 6332

EIRE

Irish Family Planning Clinic
Cathal Brugha Street Clinic
Dublin 1
Dublin 727276/727363
Provides a similar service to the FPA within the confines of Irish Law

AUSTRALIA

Australian Federation of FPAs
Suite 603
6th Floor
Roden Cutler House
24 Campbell St
Sydney
NSW 2000

NEW ZEALAND

The New Zealand FPA inc
PO Box 68200
214 Karangahape
Newton
Auckland

SOUTH AFRICA

FPA of South Africa
412 York House
46 Kerk St
Johannesburg 2001

INDEX

Page numbers in *italic* refer to the illustrations

All Optima books are available at your bookshop or newsagent, or can be ordered from the following address:

Optima, Cash Sales Department,
PO Box 11, Falmouth, Cornwall TR10 9EN

Please send cheque or postal order (no currency), and allow 60p for postage and packing for the first book, plus 25p for the second book and 15p for each additional book ordered up to a maximum charge of £1.90 in the UK.

Customers in Eire and BFPO please allow 60p for the first book, 25p for the second book plus 15p per copy for the next 7 books, thereafter 9p per book.

Overseas customers please allow £1.25 for postage and packing for the first book and 28p per copy for each additional book.